Praise for *Genetically E*

"It is great that Ronnie Cummins and Ben Lilliston have had the courage and the dedication to research the controversial subject of genetically engineered foods so thoroughly. Every aspect is covered—health hazards, effects on the environment, where to shop, what to avoid—allowing us to choose where our interests lie and, from this, check resources and make educated decisions. This guide must surely become the bible for the concerned consumer."

—Nora Pouillon, chef/owner of Restaurant Nora, Washington, D.C., the country's first certified-organic restaurant, and Asia Nora

"Consumers have known intuitively that they don't want to eat genetically engineered foods. Now they know why. Ronnie Cummins and Ben Lilliston persuasively outline the case against this mass experiment on our food, and give the public useful tools for ways to avoid genetic contamination when they buy food. Anyone who eats should read *Genetically Engineered Food*. It is indispensable as a basic primer, a resource guide, and a call to action."

—Charles Margulis, Greenpeace genetic engineering specialist

"Cummins and Lilliston are clear, accurate and compelling. If you want to understand the dangers of genetically engineered food, this is the book you need. And if you want to make safe food choices for your family, this is the book you should buy."

—Cheryl Long, senior editor of *Organic Gardening* magazine

"I breathed a sigh of relief as I picked up this book. Finally, there's a reliable source of information for consumers on the confusing subject of genetically engineered foods. In clear language, Cummins and Lilliston guide us to greater knowledge...and greater hopefulness. If you only read one book on GE foods, this should be the one."

—Peggy O'Mara, editor and publisher, *Mothering* magazine

GENETICALLY ENGINEERED FOOD

A Self-Defense Guide for Consumers

RONNIE CUMMINS AND BEN LILLISTON
FOREWORD BY ANDREW KIMBRELL

Pat Van Barneveld
1075 Ruth St., Apt. 503
Prescott, AZ 86301

MARLOWE & COMPANY
NEW YORK

Published by
Marlowe & Company
A Division of Avalon Publishing Group Incorporated
841 Broadway, 4th Floor
New York, NY 10003

Library of Congress Cataloging-in-Publication Data

Cummins, Ronnie.
GENETICALLY ENGINEERED FOOD: A Self-Defense Guide For Consumers / by Ronnie
Cummins and Ben Lilliston.
p. cm
ISBN 1-56924-635-1
1. Food—Biotechnology—Popular works. 2. Crops—Genetic engineering—
Popular works. I. Lilliston, Ben. II. Title.

TP248.65.F66 C85 2000
363.19'2—dc21   00-021900

9 8 7 6 5 4 3 2

Designed by Pauline Neuwirth, Neuwirth & Associates, Inc.

Distributed by Publishers Group West
Manufactured in the United States of America

DEDICATION

FOR THE consumers and farmers worldwide who are helping to move us toward a food and agricultural system, which is organic, sustainable, humane, and equitable

CONTENTS

FOREWORD

LIKE MANY other Americans of my generation, I was brought up at a time when we were told that "progress was our middle name," that we were going to have "better living through chemistry," and that "DDT is good for me." Prognosticators confidently predicted that, like the Jetson family of TV fame, we would soon all meet our daily nutritional requirements by eating tablets rather than food and, like the astronauts, Tang would be our beverage of choice. Unfortunately, there are those who are still committed to this decades-old "artificial is better" worldview. They still dream of a thoroughly industrialized food supply—one that depends on chemical and biological inputs, massive factory-like farms, and that results in huge corporate profits.

Remarkably, something happened on the way to this future. Despite untold billions spent in research and advertising, the public en masse has begun to reject this vision of industrial food and all that accompanies it. We have begun to understand that these chemical and biological techno-fixes come with hidden and terrible costs to human health and to the environment. We have seen cancer epidemics, widespread pollution of water and air, exponential loss of topsoil and biodiversity, terrible cruelty to animals and, most directly, tasteless and unhealthy food.

Tens of millions of Americans have decided to vote, day after day, with their food dollars. More of us are eating organic than ever before, and organic food production is the fastest-growing segment in US agriculture today. We have also realized that we are not simply consumers of food; as importantly, we are creators of our food future and the future that awaits our children and their children.

This historic clash of visions for our food future has now reached a critical moment. As this timely and important book vividly describes, we are currently witnessing the most profound alteration of food in human history. The use of chemicals and fossil fuels in our food system has had devastating consequences. Yet the use of genetic engineering is, stunningly, even more momentous and potentially more dangerous.

Ronnie Cummins and Ben Lilliston have done consumers a great service by providing well-researched findings on how genetically engineered foods could create major health hazards. Cummins and Lilliston show us how the genetic engineering of food could render formerly safe food into toxic and dangerous products, how these novel foods create new allergenic risks, and how they lower nutrition. They report on studies showing that genetically engineered foods could result in impairment of the immune system and increasing resistance to important antibiotics, and they also demonstrate that the genetic engineering of crops and food animals could have devastating environmental impacts— including an increased use of herbicides and the extinction of entire species. And they show us why the use of this technology in food production also represents a profound threat to small farmers in this country and around the world.

Despite the many potential risks of GE foods, the US government, under pressure from the ag-biotech industry, has failed to require any mandatory human health testing of GE foods. To make matters worse, the US, unlike other industrialized countries elsewhere in the world, does not require mandatory labeling of genetically engineered foods. *Genetically Engineered Food: A Self-Defense Guide for Consumers* helps to make up for this absence of information by providing the public with smart, consumer-oriented ways to avoid GE foods.

Virtually every poll taken has shown that the vast majority of Americans does not want genetically engineered foods. The only hope those who are invested in this technology have is to try and keep the public in the dark about which foods have been genetically altered and the risks these foods represent. This book is the perfect tool with which to defeat the misinformation strategy on GE foods. It is a comprehensive guide that provides consumers with the information needed to become informed about these foods. Please read it carefully and join the fight for a new food future.

Andrew Kimbrell
Center for Food Safety
Washington, D.C.
June 2000

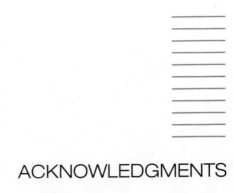

ACKNOWLEDGMENTS

MANY INDIVIDUALS and organizations helped in the writing of this book. The list is too long to name everyone. But here are a few people whose assistance was greatly appreciated: Gabriela Flora, Marnie Glickman, Michael Hansen, Simon Harris, Andy Kimbrell, Judy Linman, Charles Margulis, Loranda McLeet, Joe Mendelson, Ana Micka, Sarah Newport, Debbie Ortman, Karen Smith, John Stauber, and Rose Welch.

We'd like to extend a special thank you to our editor, Matthew Lore, for his enthusiasm and commitment to this book.

PREFACE

AS THIS book goes to press, the debate over genetically engineered foods and crops continues to escalate. Nearly every week, changes are taking place in the marketplace (where major food companies like Gerber, Heinz, and Frito-Lay are going GE-free); world trade rules are being hammered out at World Trade Organization and Biosafety Treaty negotiations; and legislative bills on labeling and safety testing are being introduced at the federal and state level. Wall Street is jittery about the future of agriculture biotechnology. Farmers and rural communities are caught in the middle of this global food fight. Even scientists and researchers are concerned about the growing influence of financial investors over independent science. And most importantly, ordinary consumers and parents are raising questions, educating themselves, and taking action.

In fact, what once appeared to be the inevitable dawn of the Biotech Century for American agriculture may well turn out to be the beginning of a serious and thoughtful reexamination of how food is produced. As part of this re-examination, we are already seeing phenomenal expansion in the demand for organic foods—following the lead of Great Britain, Japan, and much of Europe.

The debate over genetically engineered foods and crops may last decades. However, as Europe has shown, the ultimate arbiter of power in this debate is the consumer. Marketplace pressure can change the landscape quickly. If U.S. consumers are ready to take action in their everyday lives—following the food-buying and food preparation suggestions in the second half of this book—genetically engineered foods will be short-lived. Food companies, restaurants, supermarkets, institutional investors—even politicians—recognize what affects their bottom line. If American consumers reject genetically engineered foods, putting their food dollars where their concerns and values lie, this technology will fail.

We feel fortunate to be publishing this book at the very moment that public concern and awareness is growing about this radical new technology. Please read this book and pass it around to your friends, but also be prepared to take action for the future of our food. The old adage, you are what you eat, has never been more applicable. Bon Appetit!

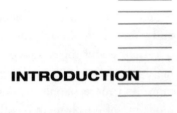

INTRODUCTION

WHAT'S FOR DINNER?
The Genetically Engineered Foods Controversy

WALK THROUGH the aisles of any supermarket in America. Sit down to eat in just about any restaurant, school cafeteria, workplace lunchroom, hospital, or airplane. Open your cupboards and refrigerator. Look at what's cooking in your oven, microwave, or frying pan, or what's on your fork, your spoon, in your cup or drinking glass . . . You can't see, smell, taste, or feel the difference. And you can't read about it on food labels or restaurant menus. But you and your family are now part of a vast culinary and biological experiment—dining on an expanding menu of genetically engineered foods. Foods that are unlike any foods consumed in human history.

Genetically engineered foods (see the box below for other comparable, frequently used terms) have been big news in Europe, Asia, and Australia for the last several years. European and

Japanese consumers have led the way, resoundingly rejecting American gene-food exports and forcing major supermarket chains and food manufacturers overseas to remove genetically engineered foods and ingredients from the marketplace. Now individual consumers, consumer advocates, research scientists, environmental organizations, and other concerned citizens in the United States and Canada are joining the debate—helping to raise substantive questions about the risks—potential and known—of this new and highly touted technology. The most urgent question being asked by more and more people worldwide is: Are genetically engineered foods harmful to human health and the environment?

DIFFERENT NAMES, SAME MEANING

Around the world, and even in this book, you will find a number of different terms or abbreviations for genetically engineered (GE) foods and organisms. Many of these terms mean the same thing, but reflect different cultural biases relative to language. Below is a short list of common terms and definitions.

- Genetically engineered (GE)—This is the standard U.S. term for a process in which foreign genes are spliced into a non-related species, creating an entirely new organism.
- Genetically modified (GM)—The same as GE, this term is more widely used in Europe because it translates more easily among different languages.
- Genetically modified organisms (GMO)—The actual organism that is created through genetic engineering.
- Biotech foods, gene-foods, bioengineered food, gene-altered foods, transgenic foods—Foods that have been created through genetic engineering.
- Frankenfoods—Another term for the above, refers to the story of Frankenstein and science gone bad.

Not since the anti-nuclear power debates in the late 1970s has there been such controversy over a new technology of this magnitude. Like their counterparts in the nuclear industry thirty years ago, the proponents of agricultural genetic engineering offer consumers a cornucopia of benefits, promising to end world hunger, improve public health, and help clean up the environment. They confidently proclaim that gene-foods are safe. They cite industry-sponsored studies and invoke the names of national and international regulatory agencies that have given dozens of genetically engineered foods clearance for commercialization. But like their predecessors in the nuclear industry a generation ago, the more they talk, and the more independent scientific evidence accumulates, the less credible proponents seem. What's becoming clear is that:

- Agricultural genetic engineering is a radical and unpredictable new technology.
- GE foods are not being adequately safety-tested for possible damage to our health.
- GE crops are not being adequately safety-tested for possible damage to the environment.
- Genetically engineered foods are everywhere, and they are not labeled.
- Agricultural genetic engineering has negative social and economic impacts on family farmers and rural communities in the U.S. and around the world.
- Mounting scientific evidence indicates that genetically engineered foods and crops may present serious hazards for our health and our environment.

A GROWING CONCERN IN NORTH AMERICA

ALTHOUGH THE volume of the genetically engineered foods debate is not yet as intense in North America as it is in Europe,

Japan, Australia, and a number of other nations, the tenor of the discussion is steadily—and now very quickly—rising in the United States. In fact, it is clear that Americans are increasingly nervous about this new and controversial technology, and strongly feel the need for additional information. Public concern in the U.S. over gene-foods is not new, however. As far back as 1994, when the first two genetically engineered foods were introduced in the United States there were clear signs of consumer skepticism. The introduction of the Bovine Growth Hormone, injected into dairy cows to force them to produce more milk, led to the tripling of the market for organic milk. The Flavr Savr tomato, which had been gene-altered for longer shelf life, fell flat on its face when consumers refused to buy it. (We will discuss these and other gene-foods in greater depth later in the book.)

National polls repeatedly reflect the depth of concern among Americans about genetically engineered food. In January 1999, *Time Magazine* found that 82 percent of Americans thought genetically engineered foods should be labeled. In this same poll, 58 percent said if GE foods were labeled, they would not buy them. A February 1997 poll by Novartis, a giant biotechnology company, found that 93 percent of Americans believe genetically engineered foods should be labeled, and 73 percent of those strongly supported that conclusion. And a September 1999 Gallup poll found that 68 percent of us would actually be willing to pay more for foods in order to guarantee that GE foods were labeled. Again and again, polls of consumers find that 80–95 percent of Americans want genetically engineered foods to be labeled—primarily so that we can avoid buying or consuming them.[1]

AMERICA'S ALTERED HARVEST: STARTLING STATISTICS ON KEY CROPS

WHILE MANY consumers have remained anxious or concerned about genetically engineered foods, a significant percentage of farmers in the U.S. have embraced the new technology. By 1999, over sixty million acres of GE crops were planted in the U.S., representing, according to The *New York Times*, almost one-quarter of our nation's food and fiber crops. The American gene-altered harvest of 1999 included approximately:

- 57 percent of U.S. soybeans
- 38 percent of U.S. corn
- 65 percent of U.S. cotton
- 4 percent of U.S. potatoes
- Over 50 percent of the U.S. and Canadian canola crop

Source: U.S. Department of Agriculture

In addition to these genetically engineered crops, at least 500,000 of the U.S.'s nine million dairy cows are being injected regularly with recombinant Bovine Growth Hormone (sometimes referred to as rBGH or rBST). Recombinant Bovine Growth Hormone is banned in Europe, Canada, and every other industrialized nation except the United States.

By the beginning of 2000, a full menu of GE foods, crops, and micro-organisms have made their way into kitchens and shopping carts nationwide. Analysts estimate that a full 60–75 percent of processed foods commonly found on supermarket shelves or at your favorite restaurant would "test positive" for the presence of gene-altered soy, corn, canola, and ingredients derived from these genetically engineered crops.

GENE-FOODS ARE EVERYWHERE
—IN MANY OF THE FOODS THAT WE EAT!

ALTHOUGH GENETICALLY engineered foods are neither required to be safety-tested nor to be labeled, they are now part of your everyday diet.[2] According to laboratory tests carried out on behalf of The *New York Times* and *Consumer Reports*, as well as disclosures by food and biotechnology companies, your daily intake of genetically modified organisms (GMOs) may now come from the following foods, among others:

- baby foods
- baking mixes
- breakfast cereals
- cooking oils
- corn
- corn chips
- corn sweeteners
- dairy products
- infant formula
- margarine
- papayas
- popcorn
- potatoes
- radicchio
- salad dressings
- soy burgers
- squash
- tomatoes

Hundreds of other genetically engineered foods and ingredients are poised for commercialization—that is, for sale to consumers, farmers (in seed form), and food manufacturers. Wherever foods are sold or served, it is becoming increasingly difficult for you to avoid purchasing or ingesting genetically engineered foods—without your knowledge.

How did this ever-expanding menu of GE foods get into our shopping carts, kitchens, restaurants, nursing homes, and onto our kids' school lunch trays? How did we get into a situation where much, if not most, of the food we eat everyday has been genetically engineered, without our approval or consent and without—at least until very recently—even our knowledge? And why have we as citizens been largely excluded from the discussions and policy decisions on genetically engineered foods?

GROWING DOUBTS, MORE QUESTIONS FOR CONSUMERS

AS GE crops become more prevalent, they are undergoing greater scrutiny. Unfortunately, upon closer examination the technology raises doubts rather than confidence. Three recent events have catalyzed public debate among the media and public:

- The prestigious British Medical Association (the equivalent of the American Medical Association, or AMA, in the U.S.) has called for a moratorium on all genetically engineered foods because they may not be safe;
- After reviewing the scientific data, Canada, the European Union, and a number of other industrialized nations have banned Bovine Growth Hormone;
- The pollen from genetically engineered corn is poisonous to Monarch butterflies.

Likewise, more Americans are asking why our government agencies designated to protect us—the Food and Drug Administration, the U.S. Department of Agriculture, and the Environmental Protection Agency—have not been more active in regulating genetically engineered foods.

NO LABELS ON GENE-FOODS: DENYING YOUR RIGHT TO KNOW

THERE IS one fundamental reason why gene-foods are now being grown, sold, and served all over the U.S.: because the corporations that have invested billions of dollars in this new technology have successfully lobbied U.S. government agencies to allow genetically engineered foods to enter our food chain and the environment virtually undetected. In the space of only five years, the agricultural biotechnology industry has not only managed to begin to transform many of the foods you eat everyday, but, even more amazingly, have managed to do so, for the most part, without your knowledge.

Imagine a pharmaceutical company slipping an entirely different chemical or additive into a well-known over-the-counter drug, and continuing to market the drug as the same well-known drug—never telling the consumer about the different chemical composition. Remarkably, this is what the agriculture biotech industry is doing to our food—they are changing its make-up, and selling it to us as if it's the same food we've eaten all our lives.

The biotech industry's opposition to labeling is not surprising. As Norman Braksick, the president of Asgrow Seed Co., a biotechnology seed company (now owned by Monsanto) admitted to the *Kansas City Star* in 1994, "If you put a label on a genetically engineered food you might as well put a skull and crossbones on it."[3]

Unfortunately, many of the current biotech companies do not have a good track record when it comes to informing the public about potential hazards of their products. Many of today's largest agricultural biotechnology companies (some refer to themselves as "Life Science" companies) are the corporations (or their successors) that in the last half of the twentieth century introduced toxic pesticides, DDT, Agent Orange, PCBs, dioxin, and many other pollutants and carcinogens. As far back as 1964, Rachel Carson warned in her then-groundbreaking book, *Silent Spring*, that putting chemical companies in charge of our food chain was not a good idea.

THE QUESTIONS WE SHOULD
ALL BE ASKING

BECAUSE GENETIC engineering is so startlingly different than anything we've ever encountered, it raises a number of important questions—many of which have yet to be answered. What exactly is genetic engineering, and how dangerous is this new technology? How does genetic engineering differ from traditional plant breeding and animal husbandry? Is gene-splicing an exact science, or is it more like William Tell shooting an apple off your head wearing a blindfold (to paraphrase Dr. Arpad Pusztai, a prominent biochemist in Great Britain)? What are the primary human health, environmental, social, and ethical hazards of genetic engineering? What about reports that gene-foods may contain:

- harmful allergens
- toxins or poisons
- antibiotic-resistant genes
- infective viral agents
- lowered nutritional values
- greater pesticide residues
- substances causing human immune system damage
- substances that increase cancer hazards

What about reports of GE crops:

- killing Monarch butterflies
- killing beneficial insects
- damaging soil fertility
- creating "superweeds"
- creating "superpests"
- creating new virulent plant viruses
- causing genetic pollution and genetic drift
- contaminating conventional and organic crops
- threatening wildlife, birds, and biodiversity

What about the negative impact of genetic engineering on family farmers and rural communities in the U.S. as well as subsistence farmers and rural villagers around the world? What about contracts farmers must sign that prohibit them from saving and replanting their own seeds and allow seed companies to inspect their property at any time? Are GE crops really improving yields? What about the claims of the agricultural biotechnology industry that GE crops will feed the hungry, promote sustainable agriculture, and enhance public health?

And are U.S. government regulatory agencies doing all they can to protect public health and the environment? Can food corporations in the U.S. be pressured to reject genetic engineering as they have in Europe and Japan?

WHAT WILL THIS BOOK DO FOR YOU?
WHAT CAN *YOU* DO FOR YOURSELF
AND YOUR FAMILY?

GENETICALLY ENGINEERED *Food: A Self-Defense Guide for Consumers* has two primary objectives. Our first goal is to help you to clearly understand why you should be concerned about purchasing or consuming genetically engineered foods in terms of human health hazards. We'll also alert you to the risks that genetically engineered crops are posing to the environment, and help you to understand why a genetically engineered future is not one we want our children, our children's children, or any future generations to inherit. Our second goal is to provide you with the practical steps and strategies you can take to defend yourself and your family from the hazards and uncertainties of foods derived from genetically modified organisms. The good news is that there is a lot you *can* do—every day—as you buy groceries, prepare meals, and dine out in restaurants. We will help you to understand what you can tell from reading ingredients labels on food packages, and what should you be concerned about when you go out to a restaurant, or when your kids eat lunch at school. We will give you more ideas than you may have ever thought possible for finding GE-free and organic foods in your local area. We will also provide you with the names of nationwide and regional supermarket chains that have publicly stated policies about selling GMO foods, and we'll tell you where to turn if you want to find out the policy of your local grocery store. Finally, we will arm you with the brand names of hundreds of organic foods and of certain "natural" foods labeled as GE-free, and we'll tell you which conventional foods are GE-free.

Many of the strategies we present and our suggestions for where and how to shop and what to buy may be new to you. You may find yourself asking: Can I really shop for food any other way than I do now? But the fact is, changing your food-buying habits is not as difficult as it might at first seem, especially as the number of outlets selling organic and GE-free foods continues to increase nationwide.

We believe that the more you understand about the technology behind the genetic engineering of food organisms, the more alarmed you will become. This book is a self-defense guide for you and other consumers, and it is a call for you to take action—in your kitchen, in your local grocery stores or at your local farmer's market, at your favorite restaurants and your children's schools, or in the offices of your local, state and federal representatives.

There are few things in life more fundamental than food. It is no exaggeration to say that we as individuals and we as a society are what we eat. Armed with the proper information and determination, you can regain your fundamental right to know what is in your food. You, along with your family and neighbors, can reassert your free choice and sovereignty—both in your own kitchens, in the public marketplace, and in the body politic. The controversy over genetically engineered foods represents a turning point for our society. We all have the power to make a choice: to choose between harmful, unsustainable agriculture or sustainable farming, to choose between genetically engineered food or safe food. These choices lie within our hands, within reach of our wallets, our forks and our knives. We hope that this book helps you to decide the nature of the food you eat—and helps you to make a GE-free future a reality.

SNAPSHOTS FROM THE GLOBAL FOOD FIGHT OVER GE FOODS 1994–2000

A dozen chefs in white hats, flanked by a bank of TV cameras and news photographers, dump cartons of milk on the sidewalk in front of an upscale supermarket in New York City, protesting U.S. government approval of the world's first genetically engineered food product, recombinant Bovine Growth Hormone. A lively contingent of demonstrators, carrying banners and signs, burst into Monsanto's headquarters in London and occupy the executive offices. Masked eco-guerrillas, under the cover of darkness, uproot an experimental plot of genetically engineered corn in Germany. Activists in a rubber dinghy block a grain ship from unloading its cargo of GE soybeans in Antwerp, Belgium. A Greenpeace truck, sporting a banner "Tony, Don't Swallow Bill's Seed," dumps five tons of gene-altered soybeans on the sidewalk in front of the British Prime Minister Tony Blair's residence in London. Sierra Club and Council of Canadians activists leaflet consumers coming in and out of a supermarket in Toronto. Consumer representatives bow and present petitions with the signatures of two million citizens to Japanese government officials in Tokyo— demanding mandatory labeling of genetically engineered foods. . . .

Heated debate breaks out on the floor of the European Parliament in Strasbourg, France as the Green Party delegation calls for a complete moratorium on GE foods. A group of Indian farmers, in Gandhi-style white traditional clothing, stand at the edge of a field and watch as flames engulf a crop of genetically engineered cotton. In front of the international press corps at the World Food Summit in Rome, a half-dozen young women, with anti-GE slogans painted on their bodies, strip naked and disrupt a speech being delivered by Dan Glickman, Secretary of the U.S. Department of Agriculture. Protesters climb to the top of the Independence Monument in Mexico City and hang a banner demanding an end to imports of genetically engineered corn from the United States. Farmers in the province of Rio Grande do Sul, Brazil march in the streets chanting for a ban on imports of GE soybeans. Several hundred protesters, carrying banners and signs, led by a contingent of of young children in Monarch butterfly costumes, picket outside a FDA hearing on GE foods in Chicago. At the "Battle of Seattle" French and American farmers hold a press conference outside a McDonald's restaurant, demanding a ban on genetically engineered foods and the abolition of the World Trade Organization . . .

WHAT IS GENETIC ENGINEERING?

THE BUSINESS of genetic engineering is the practice of altering or disrupting the genetic blueprints of living organisms—including plants, animals, micro-organisms, and humans—then patenting these altered genes and selling the resulting gene-foods, seeds, or other products for profit. Specifically, laboratory scientists use gene guns, chemical switches called promoters, and bacterial vectors to facilitate the transfer of genetic material between the cells of species that would never be able to breed or propagate in any natural environment. In other words, scientists transfer an indeterminate amount of genetic information or DNA from one or more organisms, across species boundaries, into another host organism, to create an entirely new genetically engineered organism.

All living organisms, whether bacteria, plants, animals, or human beings, contain DNA—the building-blocks of life. DNA is a genetic matrix of chemical proteins stored in the chromosomes within the nucleus of every cell. This genetic matrix is organized into a long, orderly sequence, in the shape of a double helix—imagine a twisted ladder or a spiral staircase—which contains the chemical blueprints and instructions for what cells are supposed to do, which is to manufacture proteins and carry out the basic biochemical processes of birth, life, and death. The DNA inside the cell nucleus is basically the software of life, operating like a computer program to inscribe the instructions for the everyday biochemical activities of the organism.

The technology being applied to genetically modify organisms began with research in the early 1970s. At that time molecular biologists started to develop what is called recombinant DNA technology. This new technology is a process that involves transplanting genetic material across species barriers. For the first time, scientists used chemical scissors or enzymes to take genes from bacteria, viruses, and other living organisms—and forcibly insert these "foreign" genes into plants, animals, or even humans—and vice-versa.

While some forms of recombinant DNA technology, such as using bacteria to copy or make more of a substance such as human insulin, are fairly simple and straightforward, other forms of genetic engineering, such as splicing an entire package or "cassette" of foreign proteins, viruses, and bacteria into food crops are more complicated and unpredictable.

Genetic engineers carry out these transplants or gene-splicing operations hoping to transfer a "desirable characteristic" associated with a particular gene in the "donor" organism, into a new "host" organism which will, in turn, exhibit or express this new "desired characteristic." For instance, a common genetically engineered corn was designed to carry a toxic pesticide in every cell to ward off a particularly nasty pest—the corn-borer. This new species will then pass its acquired traits on, through heredity, to its offspring.

GENETIC ENGINEERING IS A
REVOLUTIONARY NEW TECHNOLOGY

GENETIC ENGINEERING, although almost thirty years old, is a revolutionary new technology still in the early experimental stages of development. It enables molecular biologists to permanently alter the essential characteristics or genetic codes of living organisms. This technology has the awesome power to break down fundamental genetic barriers—not only between species but between humans, animals, and plants. Gene engineers all over the world are now snipping, inserting, recombining, rearranging, editing, and programming genetic material. Animal genes and even human genes are being randomly inserted into the chromosomes of plants, fish, and animals, creating heretofore unimaginable transgenic life forms.

"This is probably one of the most technologically powerful developments the world has ever seen," EPA toxicologist Suzanne Wuerthele told four hundred Nebraska farm leaders in March 2000. "It's the biological equivalent of splitting the atom."[1]

For the first time in history, the scientists and corporations using this technology have become, in effect, the architects, builders, and "owners" of life. Life science corporations today not only have patents giving them legal ownership over the process of genetically manipulating living organisms such as soybean plants, but also legal ownership over the newly created organism itself. Thus a farmer does not own the genetically engineered seeds he buys—instead he is leasing the technology from the corporation that holds the patent (more on this in chapter 4).

THE DOWNSIDE OF GENE-SPLICING

THE PROCESS of genetic engineering may sound nifty at first. Over the past two decades, many people have become enthusiastic about this new technology, and have begun to think about the possibilities of literally re-engineering life. Unfortunately, however (as we will discuss in more detail later) living organisms are not designed like machines, with interchangeable parts. Individual genes do not have a one-to-one correspondence with certain "desired characteristics" or traits, and the "surgery" employed in gene-splicing is messy, imprecise, and unpredictable. Instead of producing "superior" breeds of plants, animals, or humans—a sort of a genetic "master race"—a large percentage of genetic transplants end in failure. In fact, only one in thousands of attempts achieves the desired results without undesirable side effects.[2]

All too often, researchers end up with transgenic stillborns, mutants, freaks, and failures, with genetically modified organisms that don't behave like they're supposed to. These genetically modified organisms can act on their internal and external cellular and biological environments in unpredictable and unexpected ways.

One of the first early genetic engineering experiments illustrates the perils of attempting to transfer genetic characteristics from one species to another. In the 1980s, U.S. Department of Agriculture scientists transplanted human genes—genes supposedly associated with human growth—into pigs. By doing so they hoped to make the pigs grow faster, and increase their profitability for farmers. Unfortunately, the outcome of these experiments was not what the USDA scientists expected. In one infamous incident, instead of the "superpig" they hoped for, the pig that resulted from this gene experiment developed into a deformed creature, one that was "excessively hairy, lethargic, riddled with arthritis, apparently impotent, and slightly cross-eyed." As if that weren't bad enough, "The pig could barely stand up," according to reports.[3]

The sobering fact is that living organisms—even the simpler ones—in their internal cellular workings and their interrelationships with their surrounding biological ecosystems, are infinitely more complex than what humans, with our current levels of understanding, can comprehend, much less successfully "create" or engineer.

GENE GUNS AND CELLULAR TAXIS

GENETIC ENGINEERS know how to remove the DNA of a donor organism, and they have learned how to break through species barriers by shooting shotgun-like pellets of this DNA through biological cell walls into a "host organism." To do so, they have developed "gene guns" or bacterial vectors that can penetrate the cell walls of target organisms and deliver a payload of altered genetic material. *Agribacterium tumefaciens* is one such plant bacteria that scientists use as a vector or a sort of cellular taxi.

While scientists have been able to isolate specific characteristics or traits that they want to insert into a new species, they cannot yet precisely control the location where that trait will be inserted. In other words, they are firing the gene gun with little idea where the payload of desired traits will crash through the cell walls of the host organism and begin to disrupt its complex biochemical matrix. This random, shotgun-like insertion inevitably causes a disruption of the order and balance of the genes on the host chromosome and can readily result in random and unexpected changes in the biochemical functioning of the cells.

For example, scientists at the University of Chicago looking at genetically engineered plants from the mustard family found that two genetically engineered lines (created using the same process) were significantly different in their ability to cross breed with plant relatives—attributed to the different location of where the genes were inserted.[4] In another experiment, scientists working to genetically engineer yeast accidentally disrupted its metabolism, resulting in a 40- to 200-fold increase in methyglyoxal (MG)—a toxic substance. This study points to a potential unexpected, and hazardous, effect of genetic engineering, but also the dramatic differences (between 40 and 200 fold) that the location of gene insertion can create.[5]

GENETIC CASSETTES
AND CELLULAR DISRUPTION

THE POTENTIAL for unexpected disruptions resulting from the random insertion of DNA from one organism into another are not the only possible perils of genetic engineering. When scientists send the cellular taxi crashing through the cell walls of the host organism, the taxi usually includes a "genetic cassette" or package of altered genes. These cassettes often include several genetic components, including the Cauliflower Mosaic Virus (CaMV), a commonly used viral promoter which acts as a chemical switch to turn on certain biochemical processes in the cell. Genes in plants have their own promoters, so the genetic engineer brings in the CaMV—an extremely powerful promoter—to overwhelm the gene's own promoter system. The arrival of this genetic cassette in the host organism sets in motion and amplifies a whole series of biochemical reactions.

Unfortunately, the CaVM is such a strong promoter that it can accidentally turn genes on or off, up and down a given chromosome or even in another chromosome.[6] Additionally, there is no way to turn off these chemical switches once they're turned on, and there is no precise way to control the volume or intensity of the specific genes or chemical processes which have been turned on.

The remarkable changes posed by genetic engineering on the normal functions of a plant sometimes result in something called "gene silencing" or a shutdown of the added characteristic. A 1994 survey of thirty biotech companies showed that almost all had experienced gene silencing. A German study of genetically engineered petunias illustrates what can happen. Genetically engineered petunias were spliced with a corn gene to produce a salmon red color. At the beginning of the season, 91 percent were strongly colored, 7.6 percent weakly colored. By the end of the season only 37 percent were strongly colored, and 60 percent weakly colored. These unexpected results show the instability with which newly introduced genes can switch on or off, and the effect the environment can have on the process.[7]

What might go wrong in the host organism with the arrival of the genetic cassette? (Keep in mind this is now the genetically modified organism or GMO.) Among other things, the cells in the GMO can begin to manufacture proteins in incorrect quantities or at the wrong times, and they can even begin to produce entirely new proteins. Put another way, genetically engineered foods may express or contain certain proteins, some of which are toxic to humans, in much higher levels than you are accustomed to eating, or they may contain entirely new foreign proteins, bacteria, or viral constructs that humans have never eaten before, either individually or in combination. In the worst-case scenario, gene-spliced foods can unexpectedly set off life-threatening food allergies or even poison you. (We'll have more to say about this in chapter 2.)

GENETIC ENGINEERING IS NOT JUST A SOUPED-UP VERSION OF TRADITIONAL AGRICULTURE

GENETIC ENGINEERING differs greatly from traditional crop breeding. Traditional crop breeding does not fundamentally alter or manipulate a plant's genes. Rather, it relies on the crossing or interbreeding of selected parents of the same or closely related species, using techniques of natural propagation such as pollination. The process of conventional breeding emphasizes certain characteristics—but those characteristics are not new to the species. As we know, humans can only mate with other humans; pigs can only mate with pigs. Corn can only pollinate with other strains of corn or closely related plant relatives.

In contrast, the process of genetically engineering foods involves using special chemical enzymes as scissors, extracting selected genes from a donor organism (i.e. animals, plants, insects, soil micro-organisms, bacteria, and viruses), synthesizing or making copies of this genetic material, genetic promoters, and vectors, and then artificially inserting this synthetic "genetic cassette" into another completely different host organism, such as a soybean, a tomato, or a pig. The differences are not only in techniques and processes, but in the order of magnitude. Quite simply, genetic engineering goes far beyond the techniques of natural propagation, and brings new, untold risks.

GENETIC ENGINEERING: WHERE WILL IT LEAD US?

JUST because the current gene-splicing capability of life science technicians utilizing gene guns and bacterial vectors is crude, inexact, and more or less unpredictable, doesn't mean that the recombinant DNA technology of genetic engineering isn't "effective" in terms of giving birth to a living organism that is utterly new and "foreign." For example, when genes from humans are spliced into mice, pigs, or tobacco plants, the entire metabolism and "inner life" of these animals or plants begin to change.

COMING SOON TO THE BIOTECH CAFE

- Potatoes with jellyfish genes that glow when they need to be watered
- Super GE-enhanced salmon—twice as large as any salmon in history
- Vegetables with scorpion genes
- Pigs with human genes
- Tomatoes with flounder genes
- GE cows that produce human breast milk

FRANKENFOODS
AND CROPS LIVE ON . . . FOREVER

ONCE A living organism has been genetically engineered, its altered genetic codes begin to affect its internal and external life and chemical composition, altering every cell in the organism. This genetically engineered organism will then evolve and interact with its environment and other living organisms generation after generation, passing on its mutant characteristics, behavior, and imperfections to its offspring as well as to other related and unrelated organisms. In other words GMOs have a life of their own. Like ordinary organisms they will genetically and chemically evolve in relation to changes in their environment, and they will pass these changes on to their offspring. In addition, they will exchange genetic material and thereby biochemical characteristics with related and even non-related organisms in their environment.

For this reason, GMOs, once created and released into the environment, are permanent. They can never be recalled back into the laboratory, nor can they be contained within a restricted pasture, farmland, watershed, marine environment, or geographical space. Genetically engineered organisms are alive, mobile, and self-propagating. Like Frankenstein, once created and released from the laboratory, these living organisms cannot be tamed or killed. Frankenfoods and crops will live and mutate forever.

GENETIC DISINFORMATION:
MYTHS OF GENETICALLY ENGINEERED
FOODS & CROPS

BESIDES THE preposterous—and hazardous—scientific claim that gene-splicing is natural and that GE foods are "substantially equivalent" to conventional foods, the promoters of gene-foods and their allies in the food industry continue to publicize and promote the benefits of agricultural biotechnology. It is worth taking a closer look at some of the more problematic assertions made by the proponents of genetic engineering.

MYTH #1: GENE-SPLICING AND GENETIC ENGINEERING ARE PRECISE AND THEREFORE PREDICTABLE AND SAFE.

FACT: SCIENTISTS understand very little about the biological function of most of the genetic material or DNA in plants, animals, and humans. Geneticists use the term "junk DNA" to describe the 97 percent of genetic material whose role in living organisms is not yet understood. Research in genetics tells us that individual genes do not operate in isolation, whereby one gene causes one, and only one, biological trait and gives rise to a uniform pattern of biochemical activity; but rather, genes interact in a complex manner, changing their behavior in relation to influences from other genes in their own organism as well as being affected by other living organisms in their environment.

MYTH #2: GENETICALLY ENGINEERED FOODS HAVE INCREASED NUTRITIONAL VALUE.

FACT: ALTHOUGH genetic engineering companies have been promising us a cornucopia of more nutritious foods for almost two decades, no GE food currently on the market has been shown to be more nutritious or to taste better than non-GE foods. The overwhelming majority of GE crops through 2000—soybeans, corn, canola, cotton, potatoes, tomatoes—have been genetically altered to survive being sprayed with specific highly toxic broad-spectrum herbicides, to produce their own insecticides, or to have an increased shelf-life. This has nothing to do with nutrition or taste. And in fact, certain GE foods have been shown to have less nutritional value and quality than conventional or non-GE foods (see chapter 2 for more details).

MYTH #3: GE CROPS WILL REDUCE THE USE OF TOXIC HERBICIDES AND PESTICIDES BY FARMERS.

FACT: THE manufacturers of genetically engineered seeds make enormous profits from selling toxic pesticides to farmers. The reason they are pushing herbicide-resistant GE crop seeds is so that they can sell more of their own broad-spectrum herbicides (which kill everything green except for herbicide-resistant GE plants) to farmers, not less.

According to USDA government statistics, farmers using genetically engineered seeds on millions of acres of crop land in the U.S. in 1997–98 used on the average just as many pesticides and herbicides as the farmers who planted conventional or non-GE crops. It's worth repeating that organic farmers—who are prohibited worldwide from using genetically engineered seeds or inputs—use no toxic pesticides or herbicides whatsoever.

As Dr. Charles Benbrook, Dr. Michael Hansen, and others point out in the book *Pest Management at the Crossroads*, the only real way to reduce pesticide use is through organic or sustainable agriculture practices—practices that include integrated pest management, crop rotation, cover crops, beneficial insects, planting a variety of crops, organic composting, manual/mechanical weeding, and natural bio-pesticides.

MYTH #4: FARMERS BENEFIT ECONOMICALLY FROM GROWING GE CROPS BECAUSE OF INCREASED YIELDS AND REDUCED INPUT COSTS.

FACT: FARMERS do not benefit economically from growing GE crops for a number of reasons. USDA government statistics for 1997–98 show that farmers growing GE crops did not have yield or production increases.[8] In fact, Dr. Charles Benbrook, former chair of the National Research Council's Agriculture Committee, has shown that farmers growing Monsanto's Roundup Ready soybeans—the most popular GE crop, comprising 71 percent of all global acreage for GE crops[9]—actually experienced yield decreases of approximately 7 percent in comparison to farmers who planted conventional soybeans.[10] In addition, GE seeds are more expensive than traditional seed varieties. Moreover, beginning in 1999, major grain buyers in the U.S. such as Archer Daniels Midland and A.E. Staley began paying farmers growing non-GE crops a premium or a higher price than farmers growing GE corn or soybeans and announced they would no longer purchase grain shipments from American farmers in which GE and non-GE crop varieties were comingled.[11] Because of strong opposition to GE foods in Europe, American farmers lost approximately $400 million in sales of corn exports in 1998–99, while soybean exports to the EU fell by over a billion dollars between 1996–99.[12]

With more and more overseas buyers in Europe and Japan demanding guaranteed non-GE foods, the American Corn Growers Association has warned farmers that they risk economic ruin by continuing to plant GE crop varieties. And because of unprecedented risks associated with GE crops, insurance companies in the U.S. and Europe are now reluctant to issue crop insurance policies on them.

MYTH #5: GENETICALLY ENGINEERED CROPS WILL FEED THE WORLD'S HUNGRY AND SAVE THE DEVELOPING WORLD FROM FAMINE.

FACT: ACCORDING to United Nations' statistics, approximately 800 million people—out of a global population of six billion—are either malnourished or on the verge of starvation. This is a tragedy, as well as a moral and political outrage. But also according to the UN, the fundamental cause of world hunger is not a shortage of food in the world—in fact, there are immense surpluses—but rather that these 800 million hungry people are too poor to produce or buy the food that they need.

In fact, the world today produces more food per inhabitant than at any time in human history. The real causes of hunger are poverty, inequality, and lack of access to food.[13]

Additionally, genetically engineered technology is designed to make money. The technology allows the seed company to control the seed and pest control systems, all the while locking farmers into tough contracts to lease the technology. The technology takes away farmers' rights to grow their own food and help their community become more sustainable.

According to a number of scientific estimates, the world population is expected to level off and stabilize in approximately 50 years. At that time, analysts predict that there will still be ample food to feed us all, assuming people have the money they need to produce and/or buy their own food. But as research indicates the best and most sustainable way to produce an abundant and healthy global food supply will be to convert high-chemical and energy-intensive industrial farming—a major, if not *the* major contributing factor to global warming and climate change—into a system of sustainable and organic agriculture.

MYTH #6: THERE IS NO EVIDENCE THAT GE FOODS AND CROPS ARE HARMFUL TO HUMAN HEALTH OR TO THE ENVIRONMENT.

FACT: IN the next two chapters we will take a close look at the mounting scientific evidence that genetically engineered foods and crops pose serious risks to human health, animals, and the environment. On May 17, 1999 the prestigious 115,000-member

British Medical Association issued a report which called for a moratorium on GE foods and crops, declaring that more "independent" research is needed to determine the possible toxicity of bioengineered food. The BMA warned that the commercialization of untested and unlabeled gene-foods could lead to the development of new allergies and antibiotic resistance in humans.

On December 14, 1999, 231 scientists from 31 countries published an "Open Letter to All Governments" calling for a global moratorium on all genetically engineered foods and crops. In the text the scientists call for "the immediate suspension of all environmental releases of genetically modified crops and products; for patents on life-forms and living processes to be revoked and banned; and for a comprehensive public enquiry into the future of agriculture and food security for all." The scientists note specifically that the "cauliflower mosaic viral promoter, widely used in genetically modified crops, may enhance horizontal gene transfer and has the potential to generate new viruses that cause diseases."

WHAT ARE THE HUMAN HEALTH RISKS OF GENETICALLY ENGINEERED FOODS?

GENETICALLY ENGINEERED products clearly have the potential to be toxic and a threat to human health. But exactly what are the threats? And how potent are they? When looking at the potential human health impacts of consuming genetically engineered foods, what jumps out are the startling number of questions that thus far have been left unanswered. There still continue to be no long-term feeding studies done (traditionally done with rats) to gain insight into what effects many of the commonly consumed genetically engineered foods might have on our health. For these and other reasons, the British Medical Association and a growing number of independent scientists have called for a moratorium on genetically engineered foods until further research is completed.

Without strong data supporting safety, we are left to look at the research and case studies that have been completed—and thus far, this growing body of evidence indicates that genetically engineered food may cause toxic effects, exposure to allergens, and elevate cancer risks. As you will see in this chapter, genetic engineering is already associated with one deadly disaster in 1988 which killed thirty-seven people, and a near-disaster related to a food allergen in 1996. Additionally, the only independent feeding study of genetically engineered foods produced serious adverse effects in rats—setting off alarm bells around the world.

In the end, we are left with more questions than answers. And more concerns than confidence. Let's examine in more detail what we do know.

THE L-TRYPTOPHAN DISASTER: A WARNING OF THINGS TO COME?

ONE OF the major concerns with genetically engineered foods is that the process of genetic engineering is itself unstable, inexact, and prone to mistakes with potentially fatal consequences. A cautionary tale of genetic engineering gone wrong is the story of L-tryptophan.

In 1988, a genetically engineered brand of L-tryptophan, a common over-the-counter nutritional supplement used to treat insomnia and depression, killed 37 Americans and permanently disabled or afflicted more than 5,000 others with a potentially fatal and painful blood disorder called eosinophilia myalgia syndrome (EMS). Reacting to the tragedy, the Food and Drug Administration (FDA) pulled L-tryptophan off the market. Thousands of EMS victims suffered, and continue to suffer, from a wide variety of painful and life-threatening symptoms including heart disease, severe muscle pain, memory loss, and paralysis.

The manufacturer, Showa Denko K.K., Japan's third largest chemical company, had for the first time in the late-1980s used genetically engineered bacteria to increase the efficiency of tryptophan production by inserting genes that caused the bacteria to express new enzymes.[1] Safety tests of the new gene-altered L-tryptophan were not required by the U.S. FDA because the tryptophan produced by non-genetically engineered bacteria had been sold for years without ill effects, and the FDA assumed that GE and non-GE L-tryptophan were "substantially equivalent." Instead, it is believed that the bacteria somehow became contaminated during the recombinant (gene-splicing) DNA process.

The FDA and Showa Denko at first suggested that "inadequate purification," rather than genetic engineering, was the cause of the tragedy. But Showa Denko's own lawyer, Richard Hinds, argued in court that the chemical filtering process was not to blame.[2] Showa Denko has already paid out $1 billion in damages to EMS victims. Neither Showa Denko, the FDA, the biotechnology industry, nor the nutritional supplement industry have ever carried out an in-depth, scientifically rigorous analysis of the deadly incident.

PUSZTAI'S POTATOES: INDICTING ALL GENE-SPLICED FOODS?

INDEPENDENT SCIENTIFIC research on genetically engineered foods is rare, particularly research that studies the possible adverse effects of consuming such foods. Traditionally, the scientific community does not treat humans as guinea pigs by feeding them new food products. Instead, rats are commonly used as a surrogate in feeding studies.

Surprisingly, one of the few instances of independent research to begin rat feeding of genetically engineered foods has been carried out by Dr. Arpad Pusztai and a team of researchers at the prestigious Rowett Institute in Scotland. Pusztai's research team, highly regarded by the biotechnology industry and the British government, won out over more than a dozen other biotech labs in a competition to secure a multi-million dollar grant to study the potential impact of genetically engineered potatoes on animal and human health. What Dr. Pusztai, a self-described "proponent" of genetically engineered foods, found was so explosive that his research was the subject of numerous headline stories in the British press in late 1998 and early 1999.

Pusztai's research team found that GE pest resistant potatoes, spliced with DNA from the snowdrop plant and a commonly used viral promoter (present in almost all gene-foods), the Cauliflower Mosaic Virus (CaMv), were apparently poisonous to laboratory rats. The implications of Pusztai's partially completed research studies were far-reaching and profoundly disturbing, because they seemed to indicate that:

- There are significant chemical and compositional differences between conventional and genetically engineered foods.
- There are significant nutritional variations or protein levels in different batches of the same GE food, likely caused by the inherent unpredictability of the gene-splicing process itself.
- There can be damage to the vital organs and immune systems of lab animals fed genetically engineered foods, in this case potatoes.
- There is evidence that the Cauliflower Mosaic Viral Promoter (CaMv), gene-spliced into almost all genetically engineered foods, may be harmful to lab animals, and therefore may be harmful to humans.

GE FOODS ARE DIFFERENT FROM CONVENTIONAL FOODS

DR. PUSZTAI'S team found that potatoes gene-spliced with a type of substance having pest-resistant qualities called a lectin (transplanted in this case from the bulb of a snowdrop plant) were significantly different in chemical composition from conventional, non-GE potatoes.

Moreover, Pusztai found that GE potatoes were not only compositionally different from non-GE potatoes, but that, even among themselves, different batches of GE potatoes were significantly different. This finding of batch variation in GE varieties is also tremendously significant, since it underscores the inherent unpredictability of gene-spliced foods and reminds us just how incredibly difficult it will be to carry out reliable chemical and safety tests on these foods. As Pusztai explains:

"We had two transgenic lines of potato produced from the same gene insertion and the same growing conditions; we grew them together along with the parent plant. With our two lines of potato, which should have been substantially equivalent to each other, we found that one of the lines contained 20 percent less protein than the other. But we also found that these two lines were not substantially equivalent to their parent. This could not be predicted. It demonstrates that the unpredictability is inherent in the GM (genetic modification) process on a case-by-case basis and also at the level of every single GM plant created."[3]

GE POTATOES POISONED RATS

BESIDE SIGNIFICANT compositional differences, Pusztai found that, after only ten days, the gene-spliced potatoes damaged the vital organs and immune systems of lab rats. Whereas rats fed conventional potatoes, and rats fed conventional potatoes with lectin added mechanically (with an eye-dropper), as opposed to lectin added genetically (i.e. through gene-splicing), were unharmed. This research strongly suggests that it is not the foreign protein itself (the snowdrop lectin DNA in this case) that is poisonous—otherwise the rats that ate the potatoes with the lectin added mechanically would have been harmed—but rather something inherent in the gene-splicing process itself.

PERHAPS MOST alarming of all, Pusztai and Dr. Stanley Ewen, a pathologist at the University of Aberdeen in Scotland, drew the interim conclusion that damage to the rats' intestines and stomach linings—apparently a severe viral infection—most likely was caused by the CaMv viral promoter, a promoter derived from the Cauliflower Mosaic Virus, which is gene-spliced as a chemical switch into nearly all GE foods and crops. As Pusztai noted in an article in the U.K. *Sunday Herald*, "If there really is a problem [with the CaMv viral promoter], it probably won't apply just to the potatoes, but probably to all other transgenes [i.e. all other GE foods]."[4] In other words every gene-food out there containing the CaMv viral promoter could have unknown effects on our organs and immune system.

Many other scientists from around the world have echoed Dr. Pusztai's warnings about the inherent dangers of genetically engineered foods and the use of the Cauliflower Mosaic Viral Promoter. Dr. Mae-Wan Ho, Angela Ryan, and Dr. Joe Cummins (no relation to the co-author), researchers at The Open University in England and University of Western Ontario, Canada highlight human health risks associated with the CaMv: "The use of the Cauliflower Mosaic Viral promoter (CaMv) has the potential to reactivate dormant viruses or create new viruses in all species to which it is transferred. This transgenic instability increases the possibility of promotion of an inappropriate over-expression of genes to the transferred species. The development of cancer may be one consequence of such inappropriate over-expression of genes." Ho, Ryan, and Cummins strongly recommend that all transgenic crops and animal feeds containing CaMv be banned.[5]

UNFINISHED BUSINESS

DR. PUSZTAI'S path-breaking research work on GE potatoes unfortunately remains incomplete. Government funding was cut off, and he was fired and locked out of his lab after he spoke to the British media about his concerns over the dangers of GE foods.[6] As Joel Bleifuss reported in the January 10, 2000 issue of *In These Times* magazine, Pusztai's research, especially after he published an article in the prestigious British medical journal *Lancet* in October 1999, threatened the powerful biotech scientific establishment:

"The condemnation from the pro-genetic engineering scientific establishment was immediate. The Royal Society accused the *Lancet* of being 'breathtakingly arrogant' for publishing Pusztai's research. The *Guardian* (a leading U.K. newspaper) reported that two days before the publication of the Pusztai paper, *Lancet* editor Richard Horton had been warned by a senior member of the Royal Society . . . that his job would be in jeopardy if he published Pusztai's research."[7]

But as we have noted, more and more scientists around the world have rallied to Pusztai's defense, warning that the genetic engineering of the common foods that you and your family eat everyday may be hazardous. Vilified by the pro-biotech establishment, Dr. Pusztai will nonetheless go down in history as a scientific hero, a genetic engineer who dared to speak the truth even though it cost him his job and possibly his career as a research scientist.

THE NEAR-DISASTER OF GE SOYBEANS: ARE GENE-FOODS ALLERGENIC?

WHENEVER A new food product is introduced into the food supply, one of the first safety screens is whether it contains any known allergens. In conventional foods this process is as simple as looking at the ingredients. But genetically engineered foods pose unique challenges and questions. Are known allergens spliced into gene foods possible food allergens? And, what about the introduction of new proteins never before consumed by humans? How do we determine that these new proteins are not allergenic? The research done thus far indicates that the potential exposure to food allergens is a very real concern when it comes to GE foods.

When University of Nebraska researchers reported their findings on March 14, 1996 in the *New England Journal of Medicine* it suddenly raised the stakes in the new world of genetically engineered foods. The Nebraska researchers found that Brazil nut DNA, gene-spliced into conventional soybeans, could induce potentially fatal allergies in people sensitive to Brazil nuts. The company preparing to mass market the Brazil nut-spliced soybeans, Pioneer Hi-Bred (now owned by Dupont), immediately ceased plans for production. Pioneer had hoped to market the GE soybeans, containing elevated levels of an amino acid called methionine (found in Brazil nuts, but contained only in very low levels in conventional soybeans), as a more nutritious animal feed.[8]

While Pioneer Hi-Bred scientists had characterized their research on the GE soybeans as "very promising," the *Washington Post* had declared in 1992: "Because brazil nuts and methionine are known to be safe, the new soybean variety might not require formal FDA approval."[9] In addition, animal feeding tests of these Brazil nut-spliced soybeans, usually not even required before placing GE foods on the market, had turned up negative when looking at allergenicity. According to Dr. Steve Taylor, the University of Nebraska researcher who discovered the allergenicity of the Pioneer Hi-Bred soybeans, the failure of animal feeding tests to uncover the potentially life-threatening allergenicity of the elevated levels of methionine in the gene-altered beans "emphasizes why we cannot rely exclusively on animal-based tests for these determinations."[10] Unfortunately, the U.S. government does not require the kind of human allergy testing that Dr. Taylor performed—which in this case prevented a potential public health disaster.

THE THREAT OF UNKNOWN ALLERGIES

THE CENTERS for Disease Control estimate that 2 percent of all adults and 8 percent of all children suffer from food allergies, whose symptoms can range from mild unpleasantness to sudden death. According to the Consumers Union, medical polls show that 25 percent of Americans report that they or members of their families suffer from food allergies or sensitivities.

An increasing number of scientists are concerned that the new proteins spliced into genetically engineered foods could be allergenic. As Dr. Rebecca Goldburg of the [public interest groups] Environmental Defense states, "Since genetic engineers mix genes from a wide variety of species . . . People who are allergic to one type of food may find that they are allergic to many more."[11]

In a Consumers International position paper, "Why We Need Labeling of Genetically Engineered Food," published in April 1998, Jean Halloran and Dr. Michael Hansen warn that: "Proteins are what cause allergic reactions, and virtually every gene transfer in crops results in some protein production. Proteins will be coming into food crops not just from known sources of food allergens, like peanuts, shellfish, and dairy, but from plants of all kinds, bacteria and viruses, whose potential allergenicity is uncommon or unknown."

Allergies caused by genetically engineered foods are extremely difficult to predict in advance. There are no 100 percent correct tests for newly introduced proteins to find out whether they will be allergic in humans. "We all wish there was a test where you plug in a protein and out pops a 'yes' or 'no' answer," says Sue MacIntosh, a protein chemist with the biotech company AgrEvo.[12]

Unfortunately, animal feeding studies, as the Pioneer Brazil nut-spliced soybean case graphically illustrates, may not be adequate to find out whether particular gene-foods are likely to give you health-damaging or life-threatening food allergies. And of course these types of animal feeding tests are not even required by the government, except in those rare cases where known allergens such as peanuts or shellfish are being gene-spliced into a common food.

Only long-term volunteer human feeding studies could even begin to tell us if gene-foods are allergenic. These volunteer human feeding studies would have to be conducted on a long-term basis since human food allergies are known to build up over time. But as we've pointed out, volunteer human allergy studies are currently not required before GE companies commercialize gene-foods. As the *New England Journal of Medicine* warned in its March 14, 1996 issue regarding "foreign proteins" being gene-spliced into common food products: "The allergenic potential of these newly introduced microbial proteins is uncertain, unpredictable, and untestable."[13]

ARE GE-INDUCED ALLERGIES ALREADY DAMAGING YOUR HEALTH?

EUROPEAN FEARS over increased human allergies from genetically engineered foods increased substantially after an article in the U.K.'s *Daily Express* (March 12, 1999) reported that scientists at the York Nutritional Laboratory in Britain found an unusual 50 percent increase in food allergies from Britons' ingesting soy products in 1998, coinciding with a major increase in GE soybean imports from the U.S. According to the *Express*, "Researchers at the York Nutritional Laboratory said their findings provide real evidence that GM food could have a tangible, harmful impact on the human body." John Graham, spokesman for the York laboratory, said: "We believe this raises serious new questions about the safety of GM foods . . . It is the first time in seventeen years of testing that soy has crept into the laboratory's top ten foods to cause an allergic reaction in consumers."

British scientists have expressed concerns about the potential allergenic quality of genetically engineered soybeans for several years. British biotech expert Dr. Mae-Won Ho, among others, has warned that Monsanto's RoundupReady soybeans could pose serious food allergy problems. As Dr. Ho stated in a legal affidavit in August 1998, Monsanto's RR soybean: "contain genes from a virus, a soil bacterium and from a petunia (plant), none of which have been in our food before . . . The soil bacterium, Agrobacterium sp. (CP4EPSPS) . . . is unlike any other protein that humans have eaten. And there is no reliable method for predicting its allergenic potential. Allergic reactions typically occur only some time after the subject is sensitized by initial exposure to the allergen."[14]

BOVINE GROWTH HORMONE (RBGH) AND CANCER RISKS

UTILIZING GENETIC engineering for animals poses unique problems—both for the animals and humans. The best known, and in many ways the most alarming genetic alteration of the U.S. food supply centers around a genetically engineered hormone called recombinant Bovine Growth Hormone (rBGH), sometimes known as rBST. Approved for sale by the FDA in February 1994, rBGH is injected into dairy cows to force them to produce up to 25 percent more milk. The government approved rBGH, the world's first GE food product, even though scientists from the Consumers Union and the Cancer Prevention Coalition warned that significantly higher levels of a potent chemical hormone, Insulin-Like Growth Factor (IGF-1), in the milk and dairy products of injected cows, could pose serious hazards for human breast, prostate, and colon cancer. A number of studies have shown that humans with elevated levels of IGF-1 in their bodies are much more likely to get cancer and that IGF-1 is a powerful cancer tumor promoter.[15]

Dr. Samuel Epstein, Professor of Environmental Medicine at the University of Illinois School of Public Health, summarized the cancer and other human health hazards of rBGH in a British magazine, *The Ecologist* (September–October 1998): "[Recombinant Bovine Growth Hormone] differs from natural milk chemically, nutritionally, pharmacologically, and immunologically, besides being contaminated with pus and antibiotics resulting from mastitis induced by the biotech hormone. rBGH has high levels of abnormally potent IGF-1, up to ten times the levels in natural milk and over ten times more potent. IGF-1 resists pasteurization and digestion by stomach enzymes and is well absorbed across the intestinal wall. Still-unpublished Monsanto tests, disclosed by the FDA in summary form in 1990, showed that statistically significant growth-stimulating effects were induced in organs of adult rats by feeding IGF-1 at the lowest dose levels for only two weeks. Drinking rBGH milk would thus be expected to increase blood IGF-1 levels and to increase risks of developing prostate cancer and promoting its invasiveness. Multiple lines of evidence have also incriminated the role of IGF-1 as risk factors for breast, colon, and childhood cancers . . ."

In other words, you should be very concerned about whether or not the milk and dairy products you and your family consume are coming from cows injected with rBGH because:

- The milk from rBGH-injected cows has much higher levels of a powerful growth hormone factor called IGF-1, which is a potent cancer tumor promoter.
- rBGH-injected cows, according to the Consumers Union, have much higher rates of udder infections, called mastitis, which are routinely treated by injecting the animals with powerful antibiotics, some of which—in a nation like the U.S. where there is inadequate monitoring of antibiotic residues—inevitably end up as residues in your milk and other dairy products—not to mention in your hamburger meat.

- rBGH milk, according to Epstein and the Consumers Union, contains higher levels of pus and bacteria.

Underlining these concerns the U.S. Congressional watchdog agency, the Government Accounting Office, basically told the FDA in 1993 not to approve rBGH, arguing that the probability of increased antibiotic residues in the milk of rBGH-injected cows (resulting from higher rates of udder infections among rBGH-injected cows) posed an unacceptable risk for public health. What this means is that if you routinely ingest antibiotic animal drug residues in the meat, dairy products, and milk you consume, over time your body can become resistant to antibiotics—a serious problem in the U.S. (as this chapter will later detail). Then if you become seriously ill and need antibiotics, they may not work.

MONSANTO'S RAT FEEDING STUDIES: THE SMOKING GUN?

IN 1998, government scientists in Canada released heretofore undisclosed Monsanto/FDA documents showing damage to laboratory rats fed dosages of rBGH. Significant infiltration of rBGH into the prostate of the rats as well as thyroid cysts indicated potential cancer hazards from the drug.[16] Subsequently the government of Canada, under heavy pressure from consumers, banned rBGH in early 1999. The European Union essentially has had a ban in place since 1993. Although rBGH continues to be injected into approximately 5 percent of all U.S. dairy cows, no other industrialized country has legalized its use. The GATT Codex Alimentarius, a United Nations food standards body, has refused to certify that rBGH is safe. Even though 74 percent of Americans stated in a USDA-funded poll published in 1996 that they believe rBGH poses hazards for human health, U.S. regulatory agencies have refused to take the drug off the market, or even to require mandatory labeling for dairy products derived from rBGH-injected cows.[17] Later in this book we'll tell you how to find milk, beef, and dairy products which do not come from cows injected with rBGH.

COULD GENE-FOODS BE CONTRIBUTING TO THE ANTIBIOTIC RESISTANCE?

WHEN GENE engineers splice a foreign protein into a food product, they most often link it to another gene, called an antibiotic-resistance marker gene (ARM). By dousing this new genetically engineered creation with an antibiotic, the genetic engineer can tell if the gene-splicing procedure was successful. Basically, if the antibiotic doesn't kill the gene-food then the splicing was successful since the inserted antibiotic-resistant marker gene provided protection. This all sounds clever, but unfortunately there is a downside to ARM-ing genes.

What is worrisome to scientists and public health officials is the possibility or likelihood that ARM genes employed in gene-spliced foods or animal feeds may "mate" or combine with an expanded range of pre-existing germs or pathogens and give rise to deadly new strains of antibiotic resistant "superbugs" (salmonella, E. coli, campylobacter, tuberculosis, staph, and enterococcus).

ARMed genes may be contributing factors to the growing public health problem of infections that cannot be cured with ampicillin, kanamycin, penicillin, or other traditional antibiotics. This phenomena of inadvertently transferring antibiotic resistance into non-target organisms or pathogens is one of the prime examples of what is called "horizontal gene transfer"—a phenomena that was extremely rare in nature until the advent of genetic engineering. Geneticists call this type of "unnatural" genetic transmission "horizontal gene transfer" to differentiate it from the normal "vertical gene transfer" which occurs when non-genetically engineered living organisms pass their genes and genetic characteristics on to their offspring.

Dutch scientists found, in a sophisticated computer simulation of the human digestive system, that ARM genes in genetically engineered food could recombine with bacteria already present in the human gut to give rise to new strains of bacteria. "The results show that DNA lingers in the intestine, and confirms that genetically modified bacteria can transfer their antibiotic resistance genes to bacteria in the gut," the Dutch scientists reported in the *New Scientist* magazine.[18]

In another study, British scientists found that ARMs and other transgenic DNA can recombine with bacteria in the human mouth and throat for up to an hour after being ingested, thereby giving rise to new strains of bacteria.[19] Given the emerging science on ARMs it comes as no surprise that the respected British Medical Association in 1999 recommended that the use of antibiotic-resistant marker genes "should be phased out as swiftly as possible." European authorities are currently considering a ban on all GE foods containing antibiotic resistant marker genes, as well as a ban on antibiotics added to animal feeds.

GE VECTORS AND VIRAL PROMOTERS: ARE WE CREATING A GLOBAL HOT ZONE?

YOU'VE UNDOUBTEDLY seen or heard about Hollywood movies like *Outbreak* or *The Hot Zone* or watched the television show *X-Files*. These and a similar genre of mass-market paperbacks are scary enough to be science fiction, but many of them in fact are based upon real world events. New deadly viral and bacterial-based diseases are emerging with greater and greater frequency across the world. One need only consider the emergence and global devastation of the AIDS virus—a virus which inexplicably jumped from monkeys to humans sometime over the last few decades—to become alarmed about emerging infectious diseases. On the bacterial and food safety front, the mysterious appearance in 1982 of the E. coli 0157:H7 pathogen, the "hamburger disease" has likewise caused fear and consternation, with 60,000 Americans yearly being poisoned by the food-borne bacterium, including fifty two reported deaths in 1998. The U.S. Department of Agriculture recently admitted that over 50 percent of U.S. beef carcasses are now contaminated with E. coli 0157:H7.[20] A number of scientists including Dr. Mae-Won Ho from the U.K. and Dr. Terje Traavik from Norway have recently warned that the dumping of increasing amounts of genetically engineered vectors, viral promoters, and ARM genes into the environment may be inadvertently causing new super-virulent viruses and bacteria to cross traditional species barriers and threaten human health.[21]

INCREASED PESTICIDE RESIDUES ON FOODS

AS WE noted previously, contrary to biotech industry claims, recent studies have found that U.S. farmers growing GE crops are using just as many toxic pesticides and herbicides as conventional farmers, and in some cases are using more.[22] Scientists also predict that as weeds and pests inevitably develop resistance to GE crops, even more pesticides will be used. There is certainly no doubt that farmers growing GE crops are using more super-potent "broad-spectrum" herbicides such as glyphosate (Roundup), glufosinate, and bromoxynil than ever before. Crops genetically engineered to be herbicide-resistant to broad-spectrum herbicides accounted for approximately 70 percent of all global GE crops planted in 1998.

The so-called "benefit" of herbicide-resistant crops is that farmers can spray as much of a particular company's herbicide on their crops as they want—killing the weeds without killing their crop. Broad-spectrum herbicides, used in conjunction with herbicide-resistant seeds, are designed to literally kill everything green. Farmers like the Roundup Ready crops because they consider Roundup less toxic than what they normally use. Monsanto and other companies estimate that herbicide-resistant crops planted around the globe will triple the amount of toxic broad-spectrum herbicides used in agriculture.

A number of recent scientific studies have linked these super weed-killers to increased risks for cancer, birth defects, and other health hazards. In a 1999 article in the medical research journal *Cancer* (Volume 86 (6)), foods with residues of glyphosate, the active ingredient in Monsanto's top-selling broad spectrum herbicide, Roundup, commonly used in herbicide-resistant crops such as soybeans, corn, cotton, and canola, are cited as possible hazards for an increasingly common form of cancer, non-Hodgkin's Lymphoma.[23] Laboratory studies have shown that glyphosate causes a wide range of adverse health reactions, even at low doses. Animals fed glyphosate have experienced reduced weight gain, diarrhea, salivary gland lesions, liver damage, cataracts, and increases in thyroid, pancreas, and liver tumors. Glyphosate has also been observed to cause genetic damage in human blood cells, fruit flies, and onion cells.[24]

PESTICIDE RESIDUES IN YOUR SHOPPING CART

IN 1996, as increasing amounts of Roundup herbicide began to be sprayed on GE crops in North America, government regulatory officials in the EU raised the legal daily limit of glyphosate residues that can be ingested by humans to 20 mg per kilo—sixty times greater than the "acceptable daily intake" level previously recommended by the World Health Organization. In a similar move, Environmental Protection Agency officials in the U.S. had previously raised legally acceptable glyphosate intake levels to 100 mg per kilo—ten times the level at which birth and reproductive abnormalities have been observed in mammals.[25] In 1998 over 112,000 tons of glyphosate, the world's largest selling herbicide, were sprayed across the globe. What this means is that you might be getting more than you bargained for in your soyburger, in your tofu, in your baby food, and in the thousands of other supermarket foods that now contain GE soy or soy-derived ingredients.

Increased herbicide use on animal feed crops means that increased residues (on soybean hulls for example) in animal feeds will end up concentrating in the fatty tissues of these animals. Dr. Marc Lappe, author of the 1998 book, *Against the Grain*, points out that "Use of herbicide tolerant crops virtually guarantees that beef, poultry, and pork will have higher contamination levels of such pesticides than livestock had previously," and that government allowances of significantly higher pesticide residues will expose consumers, especially infants and children to a "largely untested and different burden of pesticides than before."[26] The bottom line for meat-eaters is that that you're probably ingesting record amounts of Roundup pesticide in your burgers, chicken, and bacon. That is, of course, unless you're buying "certified organic" products, which we discuss later in the book.

Roundup, though the most commonly used, is not the only broad-spectrum herbicide that is worrisome. Glufosinate, the active ingredient in a number of herbicide-resistant crops sold by Aventis, Monsanto, and other companies, has been linked to birth defects, learning disabilities, and abnormal behavior in the children of pregnant women who consumed foods (soybeans, corn, and canola oil) with glufosinate residues.[27] Even more alarming is the toxic weed killer bromoxynil, manufactured by Aventis, sprayed in heavy doses on herbicide-resistant GE cotton plants (and ending up in cotton seed and vegetable oils), which even the EPA classifies as a "possible human carcinogen."[28] As Lappe reports in *Against the Grain*, bromoxynil has been linked with liver tumors, spinal and skull defects, reduced fetal weight, and developmental disorders in human fetuses.

DAMAGE TO FOOD QUALITY & NUTRITION

DOES GENETICALLY engineered food have damaged vitamin content or nutritional value? This is a very important question for all consumers. Unfortunately, as the critics of gene-foods have pointed out, the U.S. government does not require stringent chemical and nutritional analyses of new genetically engineered foods before companies place these foods on the market.

Although very little research has been done on the damage of genetic engineering to food quality and nutrition, an important 1999 study by Dr. Marc Lappe published in the *Journal of Medicinal Food* found that concentrations of beneficial phytoestrogen compounds, thought to protect against heart disease and cancer, were 12–14 percent lower in genetically modified soybeans than in traditional soybean varieties. These and other studies, including Dr. Pusztai's, indicate that genetically engineering food may result in foods lower in protein quality, disease-fighting capabilities, and nutrition. For example the milk from cows injected with rBGH contains higher levels of pus, bacteria, and fat; while dairy cows ingesting GE soybeans have exhibited higher levels of fat in their milk, as reported in a study released by Greenpeace International in October 1997.

Unfortunately, serious questions about the toxicity, allergenicity, cancer risks, and nutritional content of genetically engineered foods remain unanswered. This much is clear: Further research needs to be done in these areas immediately, before we can reach a reasonable conclusion on the safety of these foods. It's worth noting that even a *pro*-biotechnology scientific panel of the National Academy of Sciences in the U.S. admitted in an April 2000 study that more caution and more safety testing are necessary before Americans can be reassured that gene-altered foods are safe.

WHAT ARE THE ENVIRONMENTAL HAZARDS OF GE CROPS?

UNLIKE TOXIC chemical pollution released into the environment, which can dissipate over time, genetically engineered crops and animals are living organisms. Genetic pollution is irreversible. It cannot be recalled as it makes its way through our global ecosystem. In this chapter we will look at some of the environmental risks of GE crops including:

- irreversible genetic pollution and drift
- damage to non-target species, beneficial insects, and soil fertility
- creation of genetically engineered "superweeds" and "superpests"
- Frankenfish and other mutant bio-invaders

- creation of new plant viruses
- damage to biological diversity

IRREVERSIBLE GENETIC POLLUTION AND DRIFT

GENETIC DRIFT or pollution occurs when the pollen from a genetically engineered plant or crop is carried by the wind or insects and then pollinates the plants (either the same conventional variety as the GE plant or a closely related wild relative) in adjacent fields or in the surrounding environment. Once genetically engineered crops are released outside the laboratory, there is no way to prevent them from spreading their altered genes into the environment, nor any way to effectively reverse this process of genetic drift once it's underway. Because they are alive, gene-altered crops are inherently more unpredictable than chemical pollutants—they can reproduce, migrate, and mutate. Wind, rain, birds, bees, and insect pollinators have begun carrying genetically-altered pollen and seeds from millions of acres of genetically engineered crops into adjoining fields and non-agricultural lands. This genetic drift has already begun polluting the DNA of crops of organic and non-GE farmers. Among a growing number of scientific studies documenting genetic drift and pollution are the following:

- In 1994, European scientists reported in *Science* magazine that genetically engineered rapeseed or canola plants were spreading herbicide-resistant genes into nearby fields of mustard plants, a wild relative of the rapeseed.[1]
- The British journal, *New Scientist*, reported on April 17, 1999 that up to 7 percent of non-genetically engineered rapeseed plants in a lab test plot were experiencing genetic contamination from GE rapeseed plants being grown 400 yards away.

- A 1999 study by the Soil Association, the U.K. organization of organic farmers, found that bees were transporting the pollen of GE rapeseed plants more than three miles.
- Other studies have shown that genetically engineered radishes, sorghum, and sunflowers can easily transfer their altered DNA to wild relatives.

GENETIC POLLUTION THREATENS BOTH ORGANIC AND CONVENTIONAL FARMERS

ORGANIC FARMERS and conventional farmers trying to grow certified non-GE crops are up in arms about genetic pollution. If your crop "tests positive" for the presence of genetically engineered organisms, you can't sell it as organic or GE-free, which means that you may not be able to sell your crop at all, or at best you'll get a lower price for it. And you may find that your crop next year is contaminated as well. In 1998 corn grown on an organic farm in Texas was contaminated with genetic drift from GE corn on a nearby farm, causing an entire wholesale shipment of organic corn chips worth several hundred thousand dollars to be destroyed by authorities in Europe.

A number of organic growers in the United States found out in 1999 that their corn and other crops were testing positive for the presence of genetically modified organisms, even though they didn't plant genetically engineered seeds. Seeing that there is no way to avoid at least a certain degree of genetic drift and pollution, European regulators have begun the process of setting an "allowable limit" for genetic contamination of certified organic and certified non-GE foods. American organic certification bodies have initiated a similar discussion.

In Britain, the government is telling organic farmers that they are just going to have to accept some level of genetic contamination. "We cannot have 100 percent total purity because we do not have the appropriate barriers," the British Food Safety Minister told organic groups. "The organic movement has to recognize and find a way of living with contamination from other crops."[2]

Of course, setting allowable residue limits for GE contamination will not solve the problem. The basic fact is this: Once genetic pollution begins, it is virtually impossible to stop. It will inevitably spread and biologically accumulate in the environment over time. For this reason there is a growing demand among farmers and environmentalists for a global moratorium on all GE crops. In December, 1999 a global class-action lawsuit by organic, as well as conventional, farmers and consumer organizations was filed against several biotech companies, citing genetic drift and economic harm to farmers as one of its primary allegations.

BT-RESISTANT SUPERPESTS: A CRISIS FOR ORGANIC AGRICULTURE

BT, THE universally used abbreviation for *Bacillus thuringiensis*, is a natural biopesticide that derives from a soil bacterium that naturally repels certain plant pests such as potato beetles, corn-borers, and cotton boll-worms. Natural forms of Bt have been utilized by organic and low-chemical input farmers for decades (usually as a spray) on crops such as tomatoes, potatoes, corn, and cotton. Since Bt in spray form degrades in sunlight and evaporates from the plant surfaces within a short period of time (roughly seventy-two hours), farmers don't have to worry about Bt residues contaminating the food crop or toxic Bt residues building up in the soil.

As with all natural biopesticides, organic farmers use Bt spray only when absolutely necessary, and they use only the smallest amounts possible to ward off pest attacks that threaten their crops. Organic farmers know that if they overuse an emergency biopesticide such as Bt, pests will inevitably develop resistance to the spray, and then they will have nothing, short of toxic pesticides—which are prohibited on organic farms—to save their crops. Non-GE Bt sprays are the most important emergency pest control agent for organic and low-chemical use farmers in the world.

Unfortunately, Bt has been the victim of its own long-term success rate. Several companies have genetically engineered a variety of crops by splicing Bt into the plant itself. Corn, cotton, and potatoes have all been genetically engineered with Bt. However, genetically engineered Bt crops differ completely from organic or conventional crops that have merely been sprayed with a Bt spray:

- GE Bt-spliced plants are designed to continually manufacture the Bt toxin or poison in every cell of their organism.
- GE crops produce Bt toxin which is 10–20 times more powerful than traditional Bt crop sprays.
- The Bt toxin in GE plants does not readily decompose.
- Genetically engineered Bt remains as residue on the food crop.
- Some scientists have warned that certain GE Bt formulations may set off food allergies.
- Gene-altered Bt builds up in the soil when it leaches through the plant's root system, as well as when the plant's leaves fall on the ground and when the entire post-harvest plant is plowed back into the soil.

Because gene-altered Bt plants constantly pump out high-potency levels of Bt, lab and field tests indicate that common plant pests such as cotton boll-worms, bud-worms, corn-borers, and potato beetles, living under constant pressure from GE crops, will likely soon evolve into "superpests" completely immune to Bt biopesticide sprays. This will present a serious danger for organic and sustainable farmers whose biological pest management practices will be unable to cope with increasing numbers of superpests.

A 1999 article in *Science* magazine (284: 965–67) pointed out that European corn-borers resistant to the Bt toxin may carry this resistance as a dominant, rather than a recessive trait, with the consequence that these Bt superpests will likely breed and multiply at a much faster rate than previously expected. This in turn could quickly render non-GE Bt pesticidal sprays ineffective. A related study at the University of Arizona on the pink boll-worm, a major cotton pest, found that Bt-resistant boll-worms reach sexual maturity faster than regular boll-worms, thus assuring they will mate with each other, rather than non-resistant boll-worms. This, in turn, will speed up the process at which Bt-resistant boll-worms will breed and proliferate.

ORGANIC FARMERS SUE THE EPA

REACTING TO the dangers of crop pests developing resistance to Bt, in February of 1999, the International Federation of Organic Agriculture Movements, Greenpeace, the Center for Food Safety, and twenty-eight other public interest groups, following up on a 1997 legal petition, filed a federal lawsuit against the U.S. government to have all genetically engineered Bt crops pulled off the market. Commenting on the lawsuit, Benedikt Haerlin, Greenpeace International's coordinator of genetic engineering campaigning, stated: "The approval of Bt plants is a classic example of how destructive agricultural practices are now being extended from chemical to biological warfare against nature."

Jim Gerritsen, a Maine organic farmer and one of the plaintiffs in the Bt lawsuit, stated in 1997, "We consider the transgenic application of Bt to be unwise because of the high likelihood that they will rapidly accelerate resistance to Bt. Should we ever lose Bt, our ability as natural farmers to grow quality produce will be in serious question."[3] Gerritsen and others have pointed out that non-genetically engineered, natural strains of Bt have been used as a biological pesticide for decades to protect crops and forests without harmful effects on the environment or human health. Natural Bt sprays are the single most important bio-pesticide in the world—with annual sales of over $60 million in the U.S. alone, according to the Center for Food Safety.

IN THE most dramatic and widely publicized GE story of 1999, *Nature* magazine published a letter from Cornell University scientists in its May 20 issue indicating that pollen from genetically engineered Bt corn crops is poisonous to Monarch butterflies. The scientists found that 44 percent of Monarch caterpillars that ate milkweed leaves (their exclusive food source) dusted with the pollen of Bt corn died. Those that survived suffered from a 60 percent weight loss. The Cornell researchers warned that their test results "have potentially profound implications for the conservation of Monarch butterflies" and that more research on the environmental risks of genetically engineered crops are required.

Headline stories of the threat to what the press dubbed "the Bambi of the insect world" brought home the fact that millions of acres of GE crops are already under cultivation in the U.S., with untold damage already being done to the environment and living creatures. Although Monsanto and the biotech industry immediately tried to undercut the Monarch story, complaining that the studies were carried out in a laboratory rather than in the fields, findings by scientists from Iowa State University, conducted in and around fields planted with Bt corn, showed a 19 percent mortality rate within 48 hours for Monarch butterflies that feasted on milkweed with the levels of Bt pollen.[4]

In an August 11, 1999 petition sent to the Environmental Protection Agency by the Union of Concerned Scientists and leading environmental organizations, the groups warned that it is not only Monarch butterflies that are at risk from poisoning by Bt crops: "EPA failed to assess risks of toxic pollen to non-target Lepidoptera [Monarchs] . . . Of special concern is the failure to evaluate impacts on the 18 moths and butterflies listed as threatened under the federal Endangered Species Act."

Responding to the Monarch controversy, USDA head Dan Glickman emphasized in interviews that "We can't force-feed consumers . . . There are certainly more and more questions being asked about biotechnology, and those questions must be answered." European Union and Japanese authorities reacted to the Monarch study by announcing that previous approvals for Bt crops in Europe and Japan will now have to be reviewed and possibly reversed. Greenpeace threatened a lawsuit unless the prior EU approvals for several Bt crops were canceled. The Bt-Monarch controversy comes on the heels of other recent studies showing that:

- Bt-spliced crops kill beneficial insects such as lacewings and ladybugs.
- Bt-spliced crops kill beneficial soil micro-organisms.
- Bt-spliced crops damage soil fertility, and may be harming insect-eating birds.

At an international meeting of entomologists (scientists who study insects) in Basel, Switzerland in March 1999, experts warned that genetically engineered Bt crops are exuding 10–20 times the amount of toxins contained in conventional (non-GE) Bt sprays, are harming beneficial insects and soil micro-organisms, and may likely be harming insect-eating bird populations. The scientists called for a moratorium on commercial planting of Bt crops.

COSTS TO BENEFICIAL INSECTS, BIRDS, AND BEES?

MANY FARMS rely on beneficial insects, birds, and bees to ward off pests and keep their farm healthy. What effect GE crops will have on these "farm helpers" is unclear. Among other recent studies on the damage of GE crops to beneficial insects, Swiss research published in the journal *Environmental Entomology* in April 1998 indicates that the mortality rate of green lacewings, a beneficial insect, rose 150 percent after they ingested corn-borers, a leading corn pest, which had eaten Bt corn. Meanwhile *Consumer Reports* (September 1999) summarized EU research indicating that bees fed proteins from genetically engineered rapeseed plants "had trouble learning to distinguish between the smells of flowers" and suffered increased mortality rates. In Britain, English Nature, the government's official wildlife advisory committee, called for a moratorium on the planting of GE crops, citing likely damage to birds and other wildlife.

BELOW THE SURFACE—SOIL DAMAGE

A CRITICAL element to the success of farming is healthy soil. Genetically engineered Bt pollen clearly poses some dangers by traveling through the air, but what is happening in the soil could be just as significant.

The Fall/Winter 1998 issue of the Union of Concerned Scientists' *Gene Exchange* reported on recent research showing that genetically engineered Bt crops are building up Bt toxins in the soil, thereby damaging the soil food web and beneficial soil micro-organisms. A study cited in *Soil Biology and Biochemistry* showed that engineered Bt does not break down in soils as readily as conventional Bt sprays, and likely remains after crop harvest in the soil or in compost.[5]

In yet another disturbing study, New York University researchers revealed in the December 2, 1999 issue of *Nature* that Bt toxins from genetically engineered crops are leaching into the soil through the plants' root systems, damaging or killing beneficial soil micro-organisms, and disrupting the soil food web. The report also documents that Bt toxins bind with soil particles for up to 243 days and remain toxic to soil insects for long periods of time.[6]

Researchers have found three known methods by which genetically engineered Bt toxins are reaching the soil:

1. farmers' plowing under plant debris after harvest;
2. pollen from genetically engineered crops falling to the ground;
3. engineered Bt exudating through the roots of the plant.

This research underlines the urgent need for more study into what GE crops are doing to living organisms below the soil.

DEADLY GE SOIL MICRO-ORGANISMS

IT'S not only Bt crops that threaten soil ecology. At the annual meeting of the Ecological Society of America in 1994, Dr. Elaine Ingham and other scientists from Oregon State University reported that a genetically engineered soil bacterium, Klebsiella planticola, developed by a European genetic engineering company to produce ethanol alcohol from crop wastes, completely destroyed the root systems of plants which were subsequently planted in the gene-altered soil. Dr. Ingham warned that if the GE Klebsiella planticola bacteria had been commercialized, an irreversible ecological disaster would have taken place whereby vast expanses of farmland would have been rendered infertile forever.[7] Following the study the biotech company holding the patent on the GE Klebsiella withdrew its plans for commercialization.

Environmental Protection Agency whistle-blowers issued similar, if slightly less alarming, warnings in 1997 protesting government approval of a GE soil bacteria called Rhizobium melitoli, designed to increase nitrogen fixation in the soil. Despite these warnings, commercialization of the Rhizobium micro-organism has gone forward.

HERBICIDE-RESISTANT SUPERWEEDS

THE LARGEST sector of genetically engineered crops are those designed to be herbicide-resistant. Yet, these crops pose some of the most significant threats to farms. There is already evidence that weeds like wild mustard, wild radish, ryegrass, or goat grass are developing resistance to herbicides because of overexposure.

As a result, in the future these new "superweeds" will require stronger, more toxic chemicals to control them.

Farmers and scientists have known for decades that overuse of a particular pesticide or herbicide tends to make weeds or insect pests resistant or immune to that particular pesticide. Now scientists warn us that genetically engineering major agricultural crops to be herbicide-resistant threatens to make the problem of weed and pest-resistance even worse. Since herbicide-resistant GE crops' main characteristic is their ability to survive mega-doses of broad-spectrum herbicides, weeds will inevitably develop resistance to commonly used herbicides such as glyphosate, glufosinate, and bromoxynil. Even the genetic engineering companies admit resistance will occur. In fact after only a few years of commercialization we are already seeing the emergence of the first "superweeds" in Europe as GE rapeseed (canola) spreads its herbicide-resistance traits to related weeds such as wild mustard plants.[8] And in Canada, scientists reported in February, 2000 that weeds near genetically engineered canola had developed resistance to three different herbicides, making the so-called "superweed" an unfortunate reality.[9]

THE ONE THAT GOT AWAY—FRANKENFISH

THE GENETIC engineering of fish such as carp, salmon, and trout to grow larger poses serious potential environmental risks. Scientists have already engineered trout to grow almost eight times larger than normal sized trout. A/F Protein, a Massachusetts-based company, is gearing up for large-scale production of engineered trout and Atlantic salmon hoping to put these products on the market by 2001. Worldwide, researchers have found the genetic keys to rapid growth in at least eleven commercially valuable fish species, including shrimp growing at the University of Connecticut.[10]

What will happen to wild fish and marine species when scientists release into the environment fish that are twice as large, and eat twice as much food, as their wild counterparts? Recent studies have already shown that (non-GE) non-native commercial breeds of Atlantic salmon escaping from fish farms on the west coast have spread diseases which have devastated native Pacific wild salmon. Researchers at Purdue University recently concluded that just a small number of growth-enhanced GE fish could eradicate large populations of wild fish. Larger GE fish attract more mates and quickly spread their characteristics throughout the population. However, the offspring of these fish have reduced reproductive capability and so reduce the health of the entire population.[11]

Problems associated with the genetic engineering process of fish has already convinced one previously interested company to back away from the technology. New Zealand-based King Salmon Co. Ltd. announced that it would bury the remains of genetically engineered salmon it had produced that ended up with deformed heads and other abnormalities.[12]

IDENTICAL TREES

FOREST GROUPS are already concerned about the effects genetically engineered trees might have on fragile ecosystems. These trees are designed to grow faster and more uniformly, and to resist pests and herbicides. A December 1999 report by the World Wildlife Fund (WWF) found that a large number of genetically engineered trees are already being planted around the world without proper safety measures. The report warns that commercial production of genetically engineered trees could begin in the next two years in Chile, China, and Indonesia. According to the WWF report, the threat of genetic pollution is high. Other threats to the environment include possible new superweeds. There could also be unintended impacts on non-target species when trees are engineered for pest resistance and herbicide tolerance.

ANOTHER TYPE of genetically engineered crop is one that is gene-spliced so as to be resistant to viruses. Unfortunately, virus-spliced crops pose a whole new set of problems. To the average consumer, plant viruses may seem rather esoteric, whereas in fact they are extremely important to our food supply. On the one hand plant viruses, especially in a period of accelerated climate change, can devastate our food crops or greatly reduce yields. On the other hand, certain plant viruses are beneficial in that they keep other undesirable weeds and food crop pests in check. Of course the more out-of-balance things get on agricultural land, the more weeds there are, and at least on a non-organic farm, the more herbicides get sprayed—ending up as toxic residues in the ground water and on our food crops.

Research by plant virologists indicates that gene-splicing may result in unanticipated outcomes and dangerous surprises that could damage important food crops and reduce biodiversity. Dr. Gus de Zoeten and Dr. Richard Allison, well-respected experts on plant pathology, after conducting experiments at Michigan State University in 1994, found that gene-splicing plants with viruses (to produce virus-resistant GE crops such as the yellow crookneck squash) can cause plant viruses to mutate into new, more virulent forms at a rate considerably higher than that theorized by the biotech industry or U.S. regulatory agencies.[13] New virulent plant viruses in the environment could potentially cause catastrophic crop losses and kill off important plant species. Since virus-spliced transgenic varieties of plants continually express the viral gene in all of their cells, the probability of recombining with other plant viruses is greatly increased.

The November 3, 1999 *New York Times* reported that the USDA approved several applications for commercialization of virus-spliced squash by Asgrow Seeds (a division of Monsanto) with little or no scientific data supporting industry claims that "wild squash was unlikely to interbreed with genetically engineered squash." The USDA made this ruling despite considerable worry among plant virologists that this type of gene-splicing could produce new superweeds which would be immune to the common plant viruses in the environment that keep these weeds in check. In other words, virus-resistant superweeds could evolve which would overrun and devastate crop lands and the surrounding environment.

Evidence that genetically engineered crops are harming the environment is rapidly accumulating. The long-term effects of this new technology on the soil, other insects, and animals—key components of a farmer's ecosystem—are still virtually unknown. But the number of red flags appears to be increasing by the month.

WHAT ARE THE SOCIAL AND ETHICAL HAZARDS OF GENETICALLY ENGINEERED FOODS AND CROPS?

THE IMPACT of genetically engineered foods and crops extends well beyond the environment and human health. GE foods are changing the face of U.S. agriculture and posing troublesome socioeconomic and ethical questions, questions that fall into the following categories:

- The social and economic hazards of GE: the escalation and exacerbation of negative trends already manifest in the globalization and industrialization of agriculture.
- The political hazards of GE: the threats to national food security, both at home and abroad, the potential dislocation of hundreds of millions of small farmers and rural villagers, and the magnification of monopoly trends already evident in industrial agriculture.

- The ethical hazards of GE: the "slippery slope" of patenting and owning living life forms. The genetic theft or biopiracy of the biological resources and genetic biodiversity found in nature and particularly in the developing world.

THE HEALTH OF THE FARM

FOR OVER 10,000 years farmers have been saving and selecting the seeds of their "best" agricultural food crops and herbs. If a plant variety was easy to harvest, produced a good yield, tasted good, did well in a particular type of soil, exhibited vigor or hardiness to survive pests, diseases, and a variety of weather and climate changes or stresses, then farmers have saved these seeds, exchanged them with their neighbors, and planted them for the next harvest. By planting a variety of naturally pollinating seeds, each with their own slightly different characteristics, farmers were able to raise resilient crops whose genetic variance allowed them to be brought to harvest. Without the work of these seed savers and diligent horticulturists over many centuries, we as consumers would not be able to enjoy the variety, quantity, and quality of the foods we eat and take for granted today.

Over time, thousands of different varieties of rice, wheat, corn, potatoes, and hundreds of other food and fiber crops were developed and nurtured, guaranteeing that just about every ecosystem and every micro-climate in the world had an ample supply and diversity of seeds and plant species to survive. Farmers and ranchers of course did the same thing with their domesticated farm animals, selecting and breeding the "best" animals for the world's varying climates and terrain. Until recently, the typical farmer in the United States and around the world cultivated a variety of field crops as well as garden vegetables, and also raised animals, who provided not only meat, milk, and eggs, but wool, leather, and manure for fertilizer.

The need for plant diversity became evident in Ireland in 1845 when a million people starved to death because a potato blight devastated the entire monoculture (single variety) potato crop planted on the island. A similar disaster occurred in the U.S. in 1970 when a corn disease or blight ravaged the national corn harvest, destroying 15 percent of the entire crop and reducing yields by as much as 50 percent.

INDUSTRIAL AGRICULTURE: THE DEATH OF DIVERSITY

WITH THE onset of modern agriculture this approach to farming began to change. Over the past century agriculture has become more industrialized and specialized with a vast decrease in the varieties of individual crops being grown. Agribusiness seed corporations learned to mass-produce "hybrid" seeds by crossing or interbreeding different purebred strains of particularly high-yielding or disease-resistant plants. Whereas farmers had traditionally crossbred a wide variety of plants (and animals) on a small scale for their own use and to trade or exchange in their local communities, new giant seed companies such as Pioneer Hi-Bred rose up to sell their hybrid seeds to thousands and eventually millions of farmers.

The advantage of hybrid seeds is that you get a higher yield, producing more of a particular crop per acre. As market forces and the consolidation of agriculture companies pushed modern farmers from polyculture (multiple crops) to monoculture (one crop), from variety to volume, farmers abandoned traditional self-pollinating (non-hybrid) varieties of seeds and began purchasing hybrid seeds and concentrating on producing vast quantities of one or two cash crops such as corn, sorghum, wheat, and sunflowers. The economic disadvantage of hybrid seeds is that farmers need to buy a lot more chemical fertilizers, pesticides, and irrigation equipment, which not only raise their costs and make them dependent on bank loans or government credit, but also negatively impact the soil and the environment. And in many cases, banks have made credit dependent on whether farmers are using the most updated technology. Another fundamental problem with hybrid seeds is that hybrids are generally sterile or else do not "breed true." If you tried saving your seeds after harvest, either you'd get no crop, a reduced crop, or a crop with lower yields and different characteristics than those in the original hybrid strain. Most farmers stopped saving and exchanging seeds and instead went back to the seed dealers every year for their supply of ever more expensive seeds. The result has been a dramatic decline in plant and crop varieties and a dangerous over-reliance on a handful of vulnerable hybrid seed types.

As Michael Fox states in his book *Eating with Conscience: The Bioethics of Food*:

> Conservationists estimate that we have lost more than half the varieties of the world's 20 most important food crops that existed at the beginning of the century. These include corn, rice, wheat, potatoes, and bananas. Over the same period we have allowed 80 percent of the varieties of horticultural fruit crops in the United States to disappear. More than one-third of livestock and poultry breeds in the United States are rare or in decline, and half of the breeds in Europe that existed at the turn of the century are now extinct.[1]

GE—FATAL TO AGRICULTURAL DIVERSITY?

FURTHER LIMITING farmers' choices, genetic engineering companies have begun to steadily buy up major seed companies around the world. As a January 7, 2000 study by the Research Advancement Foundation International (RAFI) points out, a powerful complex of five transnational Life Science corporations (Monsanto, Aventis, Novartis, Dupont, and Dow) now control "68 percent of the global agrochemical market and over 20 percent of the commercial seed trade worldwide."[2] It is estimated that as a result of a series of acquisitions and mergers, DuPont and Monsanto together now own 73 percent of corn seed produced in the U.S.

Company Global Rankings by Sector (in U.S. $millions—based on 1998 revenues)

Aventis = Hoechst + Rhone Poulenc (France)

Agrochemical Ranking: # 2—$4,675

Seed Ranking: not ranked–$134

Monsanto (USA) + Pharmacia & UPjohn

Agrochemical Ranking: # 3—$4,030

Seed Ranking: # 2—$1,800

Dupont (USA) = Pioneer Hybrid

Agrochemical Ranking: # 4—$3,155

Seed Ranking: # 1—$1,835

Syngenta = Novartis + AstraZeneca (pending—not finalized)

Agrochemical Ranking: # 1—$7,050

Seed Ranking: # 3—$1,000

4—AstraZeneca—$12,750

7—Novartis—$11,175

Dow Chemical (USA)

Agrochemical Ranking: # 7—$2,130

Seed Ranking: not ranked–$162 million

Notes: The announced merger between Novartis + AstraZeneca is pending—not final. The pharmaceutical divisions of the two companies did not merge. Under the Monsanto Pharmacia merger, the new company is expected to spin off the agriculture biotech divisions from the pharmaceutical divisions. The agriculture biotech divisions are expected to retain the name Monsanto.

Sources: Information based on RAFI research, AGROW agrochemical rankings and SCRIP Pharmaceutical League Table, December, 1999.

These new biotech seed conglomerates have a simple marketing goal—to sell a very limited variety of patented genetically engineered seeds to as many farmers as possible all over the world, just as they have done in the U.S. As Martin Teitel and Kimberly Wilson put it in their book, *Changing the Nature of Nature*, this phenomena will undoubtedly lead to a qualitative escalation of "genetic erosion" and an ever more serious weakening of plants' resistance to disease, pests, and climate change:

> Plant species in the wild are less vulnerable to insects and diseases because they have a broader genetic base to work from. While such genetic erosion is irreversible, we must guard against a further loss of biodiversity—the diversity genetic engineering threatens most. When insects and microbes ravage monocultures of [genetically engineered] food, genetic engineers become 'treadmill plant breeders,' continually forced to develop new pest-resistant varieties that survive for a while—until the pests adapt to that variety.[3]

OPENING PANDORA'S BOX

READ ANY farming magazine and it's hard to miss. Page after page of relentless advertisements for the latest genetically engineered crops. For a struggling farmer, this technology, touted as the future of agriculture, can be tempting. But taking the plunge into genetically engineered crops is not as simple as ordering the seeds. Not only do these new crops bring a new biology to farming, they represent an equally profound shift away from some fundamental rights of farmers. In fact, farmers have been caught in the middle from the beginning, receiving conflicting information on this new technology from seed companies, government regulatory agencies, and food companies. Many farmers were so conflicted they purchased both genetically engineered and non-engineered seeds in the winter of 2000 to give themselves a longer time to decide what to plant.

CONTRACT FARMING

WHEN FARMERS decide to use genetically engineered seeds, they must sign a contract with the seed company that produces them. Farmers do not buy seeds in the traditional sense. Instead, they lease proprietary technology from the seed company. And what they do with that technology is firmly regimented. For one, the contract that farmers are required to sign governs the use of the seeds, and usually include strict rules that forbid the saving of seeds—the farmer must plant them all that season, and cannot save some for next year. Additionally, the farmer must allow the seed company access to their land at all times. This last provision is the reason why many farmers are still resisting genetically engineered crops—they simply don't want to give up the rights to their land. If provisions of the contract are broken, the farmer is subject to major penalties, and can be sued and seriously fined. These contracts are taken seriously by biotech companies and are enforced to the letter. Monsanto has even employed the feared Pinkerton security firm to enforce its contracts.

UNCERTAIN MARKETS

WHILE BIOTECH companies are telling farmers they can't survive without genetically engineered crops, the markets tell a different story. According to the American Corn Growers Association, in marketing year 1997–98, corn exports to Europe stood at 2 million tons. In marketing year 1998–99, those same exports dropped to 137,000 tons. Soybeans dropped from 11 million tons in 1998 to 6 million tons in 1999. Farmers are even getting different signals from the grain wholesalers who actually buy the crops. A. E. Staley, the nation's second largest corn processor, will not accept non-European Union approved genetically engineered corn, while Archer Daniels Midland told farmers in 1999 that they should separate their crops to be sold to foreign markets. In fact, ADM is paying farmers a premium price for non-genetically engineered crops.[4] But on February 11, 2000 ADM made a public statement of support for biotech, sending mixed signals to farmers. "And since improved hybrids will mean more food and better food, it's clear that the mission of biotechnology fits in perfectly with our own. Technology is a major asset in the fight against hunger. ADM will always use it to the greatest advantage."

Illinois Cereal Mills, owned by Cargill Inc., is increasing its contracts for crops that aren't genetically engineered. But Cargill itself actively supports genetically engineered crops and accepts GE crops to be processed. Meanwhile both ADM and Cargill are hedging their bets, saying they support biotech on the one hand, while nonetheless sourcing and supplying large buyers in Europe and Japan with non-GE grains if this is what they demand—and putting farmers in a difficult position in the meantime.

U.S. FOOD COMPANIES ARE STARTING TO CHANGE THEIR TUNE

MANY U.S. farmers have felt comfortable with the potential markets for this technology as long as they have seen a united front from the food industry fully supporting biotech crops. The Grocery Manufacturers of America and the National Food Processors Association, among others, have actively supported genetic engineering both in the press and in Washington, D.C. But some member companies are starting to break ranks. In February 2000 when Frito-Lay required its contract farmers not to grow genetically engineered corn, it sent shockwaves through the farming community. Infant formula manufacturer Mead Johnson told the press in March 2000 that they intended to "reduce or eliminate" GE ingredients for their infant formula, Enfamil. And perhaps the most troubling move to farmers was the decision by baby food company Gerber, which is owned by biotech seed producer Novartis, to take genetically engineered food ingredients out of its baby food and go organic in late 1999. (More on companies going GE-Free in chapter 7.) Several other major food companies including Hershey's and McDonald's have admitted they are taking steps to go GE-free if American consumers demand it. When you throw in the organic and natural food industry—all actively working to source GE-free crops—the united front in the U.S. food industry that originally gave farmers confidence is slowly breaking apart.

U.S. REGULATORY AGENCIES

THE U.S. government regulatory agencies are also wavering. After eight years of telling the public, and farmers, that genetically engineered crops are 100 percent safe, the FDA has proposed making previously voluntary requirements mandatory because of apparent weaknesses. The EPA announced in early 2000 new requirements for farmers to guard against environmental concerns. These new rules require farmers to set aside 20 to 50 percent of their land to guard against increased pest resistance that is being caused by the biotech seeds. (See chapter 3 for more on this.) The EPA rules place a major burden on farmers to essentially protect the effectiveness of a technology they don't own, by sacrificing part of their farmland. And in April 2000 a panel of the prestigious National Academy of Sciences called for more rigorous testing and regulation of GE crops by U.S. regulatory agencies.

U.S. FARMERS GET SHORT END ON COST

A PARTICULARLY harsh blow dealt to farmers who have grown genetically engineered soybeans came in a February 2000 U.S. Government General Accounting Office (GAO) report, which reported that Argentine farmers were buying Monsanto's Roundup Ready Soybeans at between $12–$15 a 50-pound bag, while American farmers were paying between $20–$23 for the same bag of seed.[5] Monsanto claims the differential can be explained by differing patent protection in the two countries. Specifically Argentina is not giving Monsanto patent protection on their product. An outraged American Soybean Association, which has been pro-biotech, demanded that Monsanto refund U.S. farmers the difference in price—an offer Monsanto refused. Ironically, the American Soybean Association had lobbied for strong U.S. patent laws—the same patent laws that are now hurting U.S. farmers in comparison to Argentine farmers.

AT RISK WITHOUT A SAFETY NET

ALL FARMERS growing genetically engineered crops face the growing real possibility that they will be sued if genetic drift occurs from their fields onto a neighbor's land. No insurance companies will currently insure genetically engineered crops. Representatives from the Biotechnology Industry Organization (the industry's trade group) have said that farmers are responsible for genetic drift that hurts the ability of a neighbor to sell their crop. This has already occurred, as detailed in chapter 3, when an organic corn grower had his crop contaminated with genetically engineered material costing an organic chip maker several hundred thousand dollars. Once again, it is the farmers who stand to bear the costs of the technology's shortcomings, not the seed manufacturers. In response a number of laws are being introduced around the country, and at the federal level, to assign liability to the biotech seed companies in the case of genetic drift. (More in chapter 5.)

TECHNOLOGY IS COSTING SOME FARMERS

SOME FARMERS have already lost large amounts of money from using genetically engineered crops—in some cases because the technology just didn't work. In Missouri, genetically engineered cotton, designed to be resistant to the herbicide glyphosate, had almost 20,000 acres malfunction in the first year. In some cases the plants dropped their cotton boll, and in others glyphosate killed the plants.[6] In Texas, genetically engineered cotton with the

Bt pesticides spliced into it completely failed to stop the cotton boll-worm (the target pest). And numerous farmers had problems with uneven growth and lower yields.[7]

Additionally, the product is costing farmers more than they thought. According to analysis done by Dr. Charles Benbrook, genetically modified crops are requiring more herbicides than farmers were initially led to believe they would, thus driving up weed management costs. Farmers growing Roundup Ready soybeans used two to five times more herbicide, compared to other popular weed management systems. The increased use of Roundup is already resulting in the emergence of several key weed species developing a tolerance to the herbicide, requiring additional applications to control weeds.[8]

As Charles Benbrook points out, the full Roundup Ready system is now costing farmers "an amazing $68.77 per acre in 1999, about 50 percent more than the cost of [other] seed plus weed management systems in the Midwest in recent years." This trend promises to deliver "significantly lower average returns to growers," Benbrook predicts.[9]

There is evidence of a "yield drag" associated with some Roundup Ready crops, meaning that the RR bushel to acre ratio is below that of conventional crops. A yield drag quickly translates into a profitability drag.

FARMERS START TO
REJECT GE TECHNOLOGY

WHILE 1999 represented a high point in the number of acres and farmers in the U.S. growing genetically engineered crops, the year 2000 is expected to represent a decrease. The Worldwatch Institute has estimated that U.S. farmers would cut plantings of genetically engineered crops by 25 percent. The pro-biotech National Corn Growers Association announced in March 2000 that they anticipated a 20 percent decline in biotech crops. And a separate February 2000 survey sponsored by the American Corn Growers Association (ACGA) shows that those farmers who planted genetically modified (GMO) corn in 1999 will reduce their GMO-planted acres by 16 percent in 2000.

"The results of this survey are not surprising considering the level of uncertainty facing production agriculture over this issue," said Gary Goldberg, Chief Executive Officer of the ACGA in response to the survey. "It is clear that farmers are continuing to question the wisdom of planting GMOs for 2000."[10]

The Missouri Rural Crisis Center's Rhonda Perry plants conventional corn and soybeans in Mid-Missouri. "For farmers, it definitely creates the potential for economic instability because it's unclear what markets are going to be available for GE crops in the year 2000. Combined with the real possibility of contamination of non-GE crops and the corporate attempt to transfer liability to producers, farmers need to take a hard look at who is really benefiting from this biotech firestorm."[11]

This is why over thirty farm organizations, representing tens of thousands of small family farmers around the country, have come out opposed to genetically engineered crops. The organizations, including The National Family Farm Coalition, American Corn Growers Association, and Farm Aid, came out with a statement calling for an immediate moratorium on the selling of genetically engineered seeds until "an independent and comprehensive assessment of the social, environmental, health and economic impacts of those products is concluded."[12]

ARE FAMILY FARMERS AND RURAL COMMUNITIES EXPENDABLE?

THE TOTAL number of farms in the United States has declined from 6.5 million in 1935 to around 2 million in 1997. Most of this decline has taken place among family farms. Even the small number of farmers remaining in 1997 exaggerates how many family farms are left, because most are part-time residential or retirement farms.

Farm Type in 1997	Number	Percent of Farm Sales
Low production, residential and retirement	1,300,000	9
Family sized	575,000	30
Very large corporate farms and family proprietorships	161,000	61[13]

The U.S. Bureau of the Census stopped counting "farm residents" in 1993 because there were so few of them left. (In contrast, in 1900, farm residents made up 35 percent of the total population.)[14]

Squeezed by the ever lower prices paid to them by giant agribusiness oligopolies for the food they produce, and, on the other hand, forced to pay the continually increased costs of agricultural inputs (pesticides, fertilizers, seeds, equipment, fuel) to giant chemical and biotech companies, American family farmers are being relentlessly driven off the land.

In order to stay on the land, many of our farmers and ranchers are now forced into poorly paid off-farm employment, which currently provides much of the income they have to meet their survival needs. The only economic "winners" in American agriculture today are large corporate farms; semi-monopolistic grain and commodities traders; seed, biotech, and chemical companies; and giant processors, fast-food restaurants, and supermarket chains. For the rest of rural America, the factory farm, chemical-intensive monoculture cash crop model has proved to be an unmitigated disaster.

Genetically engineered crops are driving a wedge between big farms and smaller farms. The *Financial Times* reported recently that in the U.S., larger farms are planting the genetically engineered crops, while smaller farms are more likely to be looking for the GE-free premium price.[15]

A DANGEROUS TECHNOLOGY
FOR A DANGEROUS ECONOMY

IN HIS 1999 book *Farmageddon: Food and the Culture of Biotechnology*, Brewster Kneen points out that genetic engineering is just the latest tool in the hands of transnational food giants and chemical companies to maximize their profits while maintaining control over our food chain and those who produce our food and fiber.[16] With cheaper raw materials, transnational food corporations can force their way into any market in the world and put their smaller competitors out of business. With the advent of NAFTA, for instance, Cargill was able to dump hundreds of millions of dollars of corn on Mexican markets and drive over a million small indigenous farmers out of business. Gene engineers look forward to the same "success" with their herbicide resistant and Bt spliced GE seeds helping "more efficient" farmers beat out their inefficient competitors.

Just as chemical fertilizers, toxic pesticides, hybrid seeds, and factory farming were supposed to lead us into the promised land of the Green Revolution after World War Two, today's bioengineers promise to use genetic engineering to feed the world's growing population, solve modern society's food-related health problems, and clean up the mess they've made with chemical-intensive agriculture over the past fifty years.

Even a number of the agrochemical companies now admit that the Green Revolution of chemical-intensive agriculture is not sustainable. Soils are eroding, crop yields in many places are declining, water for irrigation is ever more limited, and drinking water supplies are increasingly contaminated by agricultural runoff. One billion pounds of toxic pesticides and twelve billion pounds of nitrate chemical fertilizers are being applied to America's farmlands every year, devastating our rural environment. Meanwhile weeds and pests damage or eat up the same proportion of our food crops as they did fifty years ago.

THE PROMISE of biotech crops, as championed by the industry, is that it will help feed the poor around the world, and will be necessary as our population grows. Unfortunately, the causes and solutions to hunger are political, not related to food production. In fact, we are producing more food per person than at any time in world history, according to Peter Rossett of Food First, an international hunger organization. And for the first time in history there are as many people overweight, 1.1 billion, as underfed, according to a March report by the Worldwatch Institute.[17]

But the root causes of hunger around the world will not be solved with a new technology. As Peter Rossett wrote in an editorial published in the *New York Times* in September 1999, "The real problems are poverty and inequality. Too many people are too poor to buy the food that is available or lack land on which to grow it themselves."

Genetically engineered crops do nothing to address these two root causes of hunger. In fact, they will likely do more harm than good. The two primary types of genetically engineered crops thus far, Roundup Ready and Bt, both pose potential pitfalls for the 40 percent (2.4 billion) of the world's 6 billion people that are farmers or rural villagers.

Roundup Ready crops, designed so the farmer must buy the seed and pesticide from the same company, at best produce only equal yields to conventional crops, and in some cases yield decreases. While Roundup crops allow farmers to dump as much pesticides as they want, destroying any neighboring plants around the crop—many non-crop plants are used by farmers in smaller countries as other food sources, or feed for animals.

Genetically engineered Bt crops also allow the seed producer to charge farmers for the seed and pest control system in one shot. At the same time, these crops threaten the effectiveness of natural Bt sprays, used by farmers around the world—particularly organic farmers.

Half of the world's farmers rely on saved seeds for their harvest. Yet, as we pointed out earlier, the contracts farmers sign with GE companies forbid them to do this. The biotech industry has even gone so far, with the assistance of the USDA, to develop technology to make seeds sterile after one growing season—the so-called "Terminator" technology. The Terminator technology has been highly criticized around the world, as well as being the source of many protests by farmers.

Third world farmers are threatened by genetically engineered crops in the same way that U.S. farmers are. In fact, genetically engineered crops are an instrument to expand the failed U.S. farm policy around the world. Specifically, genetically engineered crops are all about monoculture, producing one cash crop to be sold on the open market. They are not about growing a diverse set of crops to feed yourself, neighbors, and local communities. But it is exactly this kind of sustainable farming that is needed for many countries around the world.

The economic and social dynamic created by genetic engineering, the patenting of transgenic plants and food-producing animals, is leading to universal "bioserfdom" in which farmers will lease their plants and animals from biotech conglomerates and pay permanent royalties on seeds and offspring.

PATENTING LIFE FORMS: A SLIPPERY SLOPE

WHAT HAS fueled the biotech crop explosion is not a desire to feed the hungry, but rather the ability of the biotech industry to take out monopoly patents on living organisms such as seeds, plants, animals, micro-organisms, and even human cell-lines. In fact without being able to guarantee several decades of legal monopoly (patents typically last twenty years) on its gene-spliced "inventions," the biotech industry would never have invested the billions of dollars in research that have launched this agricultural biotech revolution. Following in the wake of an obscure Supreme Court decision in 1980, which basically overturned a 200-year prohibition on patenting living organisms, researchers and investors realized that they could now "own" entire varieties of plants and animals, as long as they "discovered" them (i.e. mapped out their chemical gene sequences) and/or "invented" them (i.e. performed certain genetic or chemical alterations, no matter how slight, on the natural version of these living organisms). These life patents in turn give the patent holder a legally-binding copyright over a seed or animal, enabling them to charge a "technology fee" to farmers who grow these plants or raise these animals, or a "licensing fee" to scientists who want to research these organisms. "Bio-prospectors" have now spread out across the globe, searching for commercially valuable, patentable plants, herbs, insects, micro-organisms, and human cell-lines.

Vandana Shiva, the India-based scientist and critic of biotechnology has noted: "Biodiversity has been redefined as 'biological inventions' to make patenting of life forms less controversial."[18]

The moral and ethical problem of allowing patents on living organisms is basically this: where do you draw the line? If it's legal to patent a living micro-organism, then it's legal to patent a seed or a plant. If you can patent a plant, then the door is wide open for genetically engineering and patenting animals and human cell-lines, or even body parts, or even people. A British woman recently applied for a patent on herself, both to protect herself, but also to prove a point about the excesses of the current patent system. Scientists are already talking about a major new industry transplanting the organs of genetically engineered animals into humans, cloning humans, and improving the "genetic defects" of animals and humans. Unless U.S. patent laws are changed or enforced differently, and we go back to our longstanding tradition of prohibiting patents on living organisms, it is very likely that the slippery slope we are now on will turn into an avalanche—leading us he long into a Brave New World where nothing is sacred, everything can be genetically engineered, and human eugenics becomes a technical and commercial, rather than an ethical, issue.

Andrew Kimbrell, attorney and bioethicist, summarizes the historic questions and ethical dilemmas posed by genetically engineering and patenting life forms:

> Embarking on the long journey in which corporations and governments eventually become the brokers of the blueprints of life raises some of the most disturbing and important questions ever to face humanity: Do scientists and corporations have the right to alter the genetic code of life forms at will? Should we alter the genetic structure of the entire living kingdom in the name of utility or profit? . . . Is there something sacred about life, or should life forms . . . be viewed simply as commodities in the new bio-tech marketplace? Is the genetic makeup of all living things the common heritage of all, or can it be appropriated by corporations and governments?[19]

BIOPIRACY:
THE NEW GENETIC COLONIALISM

AS WE noted earlier in this chapter, the painstaking seed saving and farming practices of indigenous and traditional peasants over thousands of years, most often carried out by peasant women, are responsible for most of the genetic richness and vitality found in the varieties of seeds and crops that we enjoy today, from corn, wheat, and rice to hundreds of other food (and medicinal) plants and crops. But from the legal standpoint of the biotech and seed industry, the original inventors and custodians of seeds and plants have no rights whatsoever. Under current Life Patent regimes, only licensed patent holders, typically corporations and research laboratories, have "intellectual property rights." Companies need

ver" and expropriate traditional seed and plant vari-
which are located in the developing world), chemi-
ally alter them somewhat, and then claim them as
patented varieties. The farmers and communities
..ped these seed varieties, some of which have generat-
ed billions of dollars in sales and profits for corporations, get nothing. In fact small farmers and indigenous people can and are being
sued and prosecuted for intellectual property rights violations, for
the "crime" of saving or planting seed varieties which they themselves and their ancestors developed.

As Indian food activist Vandana Shiva points out, life patenting
and so-called "bio-prospecting" amount to little more than a modern version of piracy or colonialism, which she calls "biopiracy." As
Shiva states: "Through intellectual property rights, an attempt is
made to take away what belongs to nature, to farmers and to
women, and to term this invasion improvement and progress."[20]

THE TERMINATOR GENE: TERMINATING
SMALL FARMERS & BIODIVERSITY

THE HIGHLY controversial "Terminator" technology is perhaps
the clearest example we've seen yet of the social and economic
hazards of agricultural genetic engineering. The Terminator technology, euphemistically described by its inventors as a "Technology
Protection System," uses genetic engineering to make seeds sterile, to eliminate a plant's natural ability to propagate or reproduce
itself. This means that farmers who plant Terminator seeds will
have no choice but to go back every year to purchase ever more
expensive GE seeds and chemical inputs from a handful of global
biotech/seed monopolies. Despite warnings from a broad range of
public interest and consumer groups worldwide that Terminator
seeds could literally destroy the livelihoods of hundreds of millions
of small farmers who depend on saving seeds, and who cannot

afford to buy high-priced hybrid or GE seeds, proponents of genetic engineering have pushed ahead with research on the Terminator. Likewise warnings from scientists that the genetic drift of Terminator genes into the environment could cause nearby crops and plants to become sterile has fallen on deaf ears.

FROM TERMINATOR TO TRAITOR

SINCE 1998 dozens of other Terminator patents have been filed for in countries all over the world by companies such as Monsanto and Novartis. Global opposition to the Terminator technology, however, grew to such a level in 1999 that Monsanto promised not to commercialize its continuing research. The USDA, Delta and Pine Land Company, and other patent holders, however, have yet to make such a promise. And as the public interest group RAFI (Research Advancement Foundation International) has pointed out, genetic engineering companies are already working on an even more insidious "second generation" Terminator technology, which RAFI has dubbed the "Traitor Technology." This "trait" or Traitor Technology will accomplish the same basic goal of the Terminator Technology by inhibiting the yield, flowering, or reproduction of GE crops unless they are sprayed or treated with the proprietary chemicals of the Traitor Technology patent holders. This Traitor Technology not only guarantees that farmers will have to return to the seed companies each year, but that their chemical inputs will have a guaranteed market.

BIOETHICS: PATENTING & GENETICALLY ENGINEERING ANIMALS

THE GENETIC engineering and patenting of animals reduces sentient living creatures to the status of manufactured products and will result in a escalation of the already institutionalized cruelty of industrialized factory farming. In January 1994, the USDA announced that scientists had completed genetic "road maps" for cattle and pigs, a precursor to ever more experimentation on live animals. In addition to the cruelty inherent in such experimentation (the "mistakes" are born with painful deformities, crippled, blind, and so on), these "manufactured" creatures have no greater value to their "creators" than mechanical inventions. Animals genetically engineered for use in laboratories, such as the infamous "Harvard mouse" which contains a human cancer-causing gene that will be passed down to all succeeding generations, were created to suffer. A purely reductionist science, biotechnology reduces all life to bits of information (genetic code) that can be arranged and rearranged at whim. Stripped of their integrity and sacred qualities, animals who are merely objects to their "inventors" will be treated as such. Currently, hundreds of genetically engineered "freak" animals are awaiting patent approval from the federal government. One can only wonder, after the wholesale gene-altering and patenting of animals, will GE "designer babies" be next?

Aside from scientific questions, it is clear that genetically engineered crops represent a sea change in the way we look at agriculture. And if genetically engineered crops become the dominant form of agriculture, they will change the agri-economy forever. The technology also raises uncomfortable ethical and moral questions about tampering with genetic codes. In the end, there appears to be little consideration of the monumental ethical and moral impacts genetic engineering has on the world.

HOW ARE GENETICALLY ENGINEERED FOODS REGULATED IN THE U.S. AND WORLDWIDE?

THERE IS a stark difference between the approach U.S. regulatory agencies take toward genetically engineered foods and the policies of most other industrialized countries. In a nutshell, U.S. agencies treat genetically engineered foods no differently than other foods—requiring neither mandatory safety testing nor labeling. Other nations have followed an approach more consistent with "The Precautionary Principle"—which states that when there is scientific uncertainty on the effects of a new technology, the technology must be proven safe before it enters the marketplace.

For example, France placed an immediate moratorium on growing certain types of genetically engineered Bt crops after Cornell University researchers found that pollen from gene-altered corn was toxic to the Monarch butterfly (see chapter 3 for more details). Germany pulled Novartis Bt corn off the market after it determined that antibiotic resistance genes used in the crop could effect the use of antibiotics in that country.

Globally, the United Nation's Food and Agriculture Organization utilized the precautionary principle when it urged caution in March 2000 on GE crops because of unanswered questions about environmental and human health effects. The European Union (EU) has taken the lead in emphasizing precautionary measures when regulating genetically engineered foods and crops. In June 1999, the European Environment Ministers declared a de facto moratorium on the market approval of new genetically engineered foods in Europe until further safety testing has been completed. The EU has not approved a new genetically engineered crop or food since April 1998. And in January 2000, the EU agreed to label all processed foods that contain at least 1 percent of genetically engineered soybean or corn. This policy applies to all fifteen EU member nations.

Before looking at the U.S. regulatory system for genetically engineered foods, you might find it helpful to read about policies and company actions in other countries:

UNITED KINGDOM

THE UNITED Kingdom has currently placed a three-year moratorium on the commercial planting of genetically engineered crops—pending additional scientific research on the environmental and human health effects. The U.K. is also the only country that requires the labeling of genetically engineered food in restaurants. Local authorities from Kent, Surrey, Oxfordshire, North Tyneside, Southampton, and Lodon's Lambeth have banned genetically engineered foods from their schools. All of Britain's major supermarkets have banned genetically engineered ingredients from their brand name products, and supermarkets Tesco, Iceland, and Sainsbury are now making efforts to stock only meat and poultry that has not been fed genetically engineered crops.[1]

Even Prince Charles has stepped into the fray: " . . . the capacity of GM technology to change our world has brought us to a crossroads of fundamental importance. Are we going to allow the industrialisation of Life itself, redesigning the natural world for the sake of convenience and embarking on an Orwellian future? And, if we do, will there eventually be a price to pay? Or should we be adopting a gentler, more considered approach, seeking always to work with the grain of Nature in making better, more sustainable use of what we have, for the long-term benefit of mankind as a whole?"[2] *Good for you Charlie!*

AUSTRIA

AUSTRIA BANNED the import of genetically engineered Bt corn produced by Novartis and Monsanto in 1997. The Austrian government has been active within the European Union in opposing genetically engineered foods after a 1997 People's Petition gathered the signature of 1.2 million Austrians—approximately 25 percent of the electorate—calling for a ban on genetically engineered crops and foods. All of Austria's main supermarket chains have taken genetically engineered products off their shelves, and major meat companies are implementing a ban on genetically engineered ingredients in animal foods.

FRANCE

FRANCE HAS pressured the EU to suspend the approval process for new strains of genetically engineered crops until further regulations can be written. In addition, France actively advocated for the EU's current labeling system. In November 1998, the French government banned the import and sale of two genetically engineered oilseed rape crops. France's largest supermarket chain,

Carrefour, has taken genetically engineered foods off the market, while major French poultry and meat companies are also implementing bans on GE-derived animal feeds.

GERMANY

IN FEBRUARY 2000, German Health Minister Andrea Fischer ordered a ban on cultivation of genetically engineered corn in Germany, stating concerns about the presence of antibiotic-resistant marker genes and their impact on the effectiveness of antibiotics in humans. Major food manufacturers, baby food companies, and supermarket chains have banned genetically engineered foods and ingredients in the wake of a major consumer campaign led by Greenpeace and other environmental groups.

GREECE

IN APRIL 1999, the Greek Environmental Ministry blocked the approval of seven GE crops, including cotton and corn varieties. Previously, the Greek Ministry banned the import of genetically engineered rapeseed or canola, and the Greece Environment Minister announced that applications for all experimental plantings of genetically engineered crops will be rejected.

ITALY

THE ITALIAN government in December 1999 announced at least a temporary ban on seven genetically engineered foods and crops, including Bt corn and herbicide-resistant corn and rapeseed (canola), stating that it was not possible to guarantee that genetic alteration of foods was safe.

CZECHOSLOVAKIA

THE CZECH government announced in late 1999 that all genetically engineered foods and crops would have to be labeled and certified as being safe before being grown or imported into the country.

SWITZERLAND

IN APRIL 1999, the Swiss Federal Environmental Agency rejected applications for field trials of GE corn and potatoes, stating that the safety of the genetically engineered corn for human health and the environment cannot be demonstrated with the current scientific evidence and experience. Switzerland is also the first country in Europe to set a limit for genetic contamination, which went into effect in July 1999. Under Swiss seed market laws, "technical" contamination with seed from weed and other varieties can be as high as 5 percent respectively. The Swiss government has now set a 1 percent tolerance standard for genetic contamination of food. This has lead to Swiss supermarket chains and food manufacturers such as Nestle, under heavy pressure from consumers, to ban genetically engineered ingredients in their products, as has the country's leading airline, SwissAir, which now serves organic food on all its flights.

NORWAY

NORWAY, WHICH is not a formal member of the European Union, is the only country in Europe to implement a blanket ban on all genetically engineered foods and crops.

SPAIN

SPAIN'S LARGEST supermarket chain, Pryca, announced in May 1999 a ban on genetically engineered foods. Marks and Spencer, Burger King, and Nestle had previously made similar announcements for their products in Spain.

SWEDEN

LEADING SUPERMARKETS and food manufacturers announced in February 1999 a policy of mandatory labeling for all genetically engineered foods, food ingredients, and cooking oils, although most of these companies have already banned genetically engineered ingredients from their brand-name products.

AUSTRALIA/NEW ZEALAND

IN DECEMBER 1998, the Australia-New Zealand Food Standards Council called for mandatory labeling of GE food.

BRAZIL

IN MARCH 1999, Brazil's second-largest soybean growing state, Rio Grande do Sul, announced its intention to ban the planting of genetically engineered crops. In June 1999, the Sixth Federal Court of Brasilia decided that Monsanto needed to complete an enviromental impact assessment before any commercialization of genetically engineered soybean seeds would be approved. A previous court decision set specific labeling requirements for genetically engineered products in Brazil. Brazil now exports major quantities of "GE-free" soybeans to Europe.

JAPAN

IN DECEMBER 1999, Japan's Ministry of Health and Welfare (MHW) announced that tests on the potential health risks of genetically engineered foods will be mandatory beginning April 2001. Currently, such tests are voluntary. The Japanese Agriculture Ministry will require mandatory labeling of 28 foods for genetically modified ingredients starting in April 2001. Japan's two biggest breweries, Kirin and Asahi, have said they will no longer use U.S. gene-altered corn in their products. Ajinomoto, Japan's largest food-additive manufacturer, has said it will stop using genetically engineered soybeans in its products. Many grocery chains, like Jusco, are already labeling genetically engineered ingredients.

KOREA

THE GOVERNMENT plans to require labeling of engineered foods when the product contains more than 3 percent of gene-spliced strains. Beginning in July 2001, food items requiring labeling will include tofu, soybeans, and corn flour and six other grains and processed foods. The requirements will expand to potatoes in 2002 and to rapeseed and cotton in the future.

MEXICO

MEXICO'S LARGEST tortilla manufacturer, Maseca, announced in 1999 that they were banning GE corn from their products. Government officials, under pressure from farm and environmental groups, had earlier declared that imports of genetically engineered corn from the U.S. would no longer be permitted—despite lab tests by Greenpeace showing widespread imports of genetically engineered corn from the U.S.

In the age of globalization, international trade rules regarding new technologies have become more and more critical. Because different countries are regulating genetically engineered foods differently, the establishment of common trade rules has been very difficult. In fact, establishing trade rules for genetically engineered foods is one of the most contentious international issue and often pits the U.S. government against much of the rest of the world. Genetically engineered foods were a major source of protests at the now infamous World Trade Organization (WTO) meeting in Seattle in early December 1999.

Establishing international rules for genetically engineered foods is taking two tracks: one is through the WTO, and the other is through the United Nations (UN) Biosafety Protocol negotiations.

The WTO sets the rules for trade for its 135 nation participants. At the WTO meeting in Seattle, U.S. trade negotiators tried to open foreign markets for U.S. grown genetically engineered crops. The U.S. trade team viewed many of the policies of foreign governments outlined in this chapter as unfair barriers to trade. However, other countries (including the European Union, Japan, and India) disagreed and a compromise could not be worked out. The U.S. and other countries will try again at future WTO meetings to set international trade rules that encourage the trade of genetically engineered crops.

There has been more progress made within the UN's Biosafety Protocol. In February 2000, governments from around the world reached agreement on the first treaty governing genetically engineered crops. In a major victory for those fighting genetically engineered foods around the world, the treaty acknowledges the importance of the "precautionary principle"—which states that these new foods can be rejected by other countries if there are unanswered scientific questions pending their safety. The Protocol for the first time establishes on an international level that genetically engineered foods are distinct and different, and should be regulated differently than conventional foods. And under the treaty, shipments containing genetically engineered commodities must be labeled that they "may contain" genetically modified organisms.

While the Biosafety agreement was considered a good first step by many environmentalists, it is expected that large agricultural interests will challenge any countries that reject genetically engineered commodities through the World Trade Organization. The Biosafety Protocol does not override rules and obligations established under the WTO.

HOW DOES THE U.S. REGULATE GENETICALLY ENGINEERED FOODS?

IN 1992, the Food and Drug Administration (FDA) issued a "Statement of Policy" that would forever change your food supply. The FDA initiative determined that genetically engineered foods were "substantially similar" to conventional crops, and thus were not required to be labeled or undergo special safety testing before they entered the marketplace.

The 1992 FDA policy opened the floodgates for nearly fifty different genetically engineered organisms to become part of the foods we eat every day—including over half of soybeans and a third of the corn crop. Other rapidly growing engineered crops include canola, cotton, potatoes, tomatoes, and sweet peppers.

Three agencies currently regulate genetically engineered products—the FDA (regulating food and drugs), U.S. Environmental Protection Agency (regulating pesticides) and U.S. Department of Agriculture (regulating farm production). Critics of the U.S. system argue that it utilizes outdated regulatory statutes designed to regulate non-GE foods and crops. The U.S. Congress has yet to pass a regulatory statute that deals specifically with the unique threats posed by genetically engineered crops and foods.

ARE GENETICALLY ENGINEERED FOODS TESTED FOR HUMAN HEALTH RISKS?

AS WE'VE mentioned previously, genetically engineered foods in the U.S. are not required to be undergo specific safety tests prior to entering the market. While food additives are subjected to a rigorous round of testing, meeting the standard of "a reasonable certainty of no harm," the FDA has determined that the genetically engineered foods currently on the market do not qualify as additives.

Under the Food Drug and Cosmetic Act (FDCA) of 1958, if foods are "Generally Regarded As Safe" (GRAS) they are exempt from pre-market review. The FDA has determined that genetically engineered foods introduced thus far fit the GRAS category.

When a biotech firm submits a new product for approval, the company is "encouraged" to participate in the FDA's "voluntary" consultation process. As the FDA points out, every company that has placed a genetically engineered food product on the market has participated in the consultation process. But each company voluntarily submits different types of tests—and only the summary of the data, not the entire studies, are sent to the FDA. The tests are neither peer reviewed nor made available for public scrutiny. And the testing is largely done by the company seeking guidance from the agency. In April 2000, the FDA announced new proposed rules for regulating genetically engineered foods that essentially made the previous "voluntary" process mandatory. The new rules are receiving public comments, after which the FDA will issue the final rules. The new proposed rules offer little new requirements from the old system—they still do not require mandatory compositional analysis, animal feeding tests, and long-term volunteer human feeding studies.[3]

As detailed in chapter 2, a particular health concern is the potential exposure to food allergens. Although the FDA co-sponsored a scientific meeting on food allergies in genetically engineered foods in 1994, the agency has yet to develop and publish guidance to industry on how to assess the allergenic potential of new proteins.

"Most proteins added to foods via genetic engineering cannot be tested for allergenicity. Instead, industry scientists simply screen the biochemical characteristics of proteins to see if they are consistent with the characteristics associated with allergens. It remains to be seen how effective such screening will be in protecting public health," Dr. Rebecca Goldburg told an FDA panel in November 1999.[4]

Another concern is the lack of toxicity testing. Dr. Puztai's important rat study (again, see chapter 2) with a strain of genetically engineered potato is one of the few rat animal feeding studies conducted on genetically engineered foods. "Currently, there is no requirement of toxicity testing to ensure genetically engineered substances are safe—what is needed is long-term rats studies," according to Jean Halloran, of the Consumers Union.[5]

There is also no FDA screen for imported genetically engineered foods. Genetically engineered foods from other countries with even less regulations in place than the U.S., such as Argentina, Mexico, and China may not have undergone any safety review before entering the U.S. "We have no clue about imported food," says Halloran. "There are active programs in many other countries—and will be more soon. They are growing everything there."[6]

CONTROVERSY WITHIN THE FDA OVER ITS 1992 POLICY

WHEN THE FDA announced its 1992 policy, the agency argued that it was supported by a clear scientific consensus that genetically engineered crops were "substantially equivalent" to other crops. But as documents made public as a result of a recent lawsuit indicate, many of the FDA's own scientists strongly disagreed with the policy.

In a memo to FDA Biotechnology Coordinator James Maryanski in 1992, FDA compliance officer Dr. Linda Kahl argued that genetically engineered crops and traditional crops were not the same. "The process of genetic engineering and traditional breeding are different, and according to the technical experts in the agency, they lead to different risks," Dr. Kahl wrote.[7]

In a separate memorandum, Dr. Louis Pribyl, an FDA microbiologist, commented that a draft of the FDA policy "read very pro-industry, especially in the area of unintended effects." It is "industry's pet idea that there are no unintended effects that will raise the FDA.'s level of concern." But time and again, Prybil wrote, "there is no data to back up their contention."[8]

IS THE ENVIRONMENT BEING PROTECTED?

THE U.S. Environmental Protection Agency is in charge of protecting the environment from potential adverse effects of genetically engineered crops. But the agency has been sharply criticized by environmental groups and leading scientists for ignoring important environmental statutes, and allowing genetically engineered crops into the fields with little information on possible adverse environmental effects.

In a rare move, even an EPA scientific advisory panel told the agency in February 2000 that it needs to strengthen its oversight of new genetically engineered crops to ensure that they aren't harmful to insects and butterflies, including the Monarch butterfly. The advisory panel, an independent, peer review body, told the EPA that the crops should be tested on a wider variety of insects to determine their effects and that the EPA should require more data from seed companies on the impact of crops in the field. Registrations for the Bt corn and a similar variety of cotton will expire next year, and the scientists will be asked to make specific recommendations on them.[9]

For example, the Cornell University study on the Monarch butterfly, and the New York University study on the engineered Bt remaining toxic in the soil (see chapter 3)—both clearly important studies with serious implications—were not required to be done at all, let alone before the crops they studied enter the marketplace.

As we discussed in chapter 3, the EPA is currently being sued by Greenpeace, the Center for Food Safety, and numerous other environmental groups and organic farmers because of the way it has regulated crops with the genetically engineered (Bt) spliced into it. Among several charges, the lawsuit claims that the EPA has ignored the Federal Fungicide, Insecticide and Rodenticide Act (FIFRA) and the National Environmental Policy Act (NEPA) by allowing Bt plants on the market.[10]

The lawsuit charges that the EPA has allowed genetically engineered Bt plants to enter the market despite recent research indicating that these engineered plants will: speed up the development of pest resistance to natural Bt sprays (an important tool for organic farmers); transfer engineered Bt traits to like-weeds creating so-called "Superweeds"; and have adverse impacts on beneficial insects and other non-target organizations. In addition, the EPA has ignored a requirement under NEPA to prepare an environmental impact statement that analyzes the environmental, socio-economic, and cumulative impacts of its program registering genetically engineered Bt plants.

The registrations for the current wave of engineered Bt crops expire in 2001. The EPA will need to evaluate the next round of genetically engineered Bt corn—which are expected to be one, two, or three orders of magnitude more powerful than existing varieties. The new varieties will be designed to address the corn rootworm complex, a particularly stubborn pest which has developed a resistance to every single pest tool including crop rotation, according to Dr. Charles Benbrook, former chair of the National Research Council's Agriculture Committee. "It's going to take a pretty high level of Bt to control them."[11]

THE EPA'S RESISTANCE
TO PEST RESISTANCE

ALTHOUGH GENETICALLY engineered Bt crops have been planted commercially in U.S. fields since 1995, it took the agency five years to put together guidelines for farmers to address the potentially catastrophic effects of pest resistance. Both the biotech industry and the EPA recognize that genetically engineered Bt crops will speed up the development of resistance to Bt by the major target pests—the pink boll-worm (cotton) and the corn-borer (corn)—in as few as three years (as we further detail in chapter 3). Pest resistance could mean a new strain of "superbugs" able to withstand pesticides.

Under current EPA rules, most farmers planting GE Bt corn are required to plant 20–25 percent of their crop as non-Bt corn—creating a kind of refuge. Farmers planting genetically engineered Bt cotton are required to plant 4–20 percent of non-engineered cotton. The EPA hopes that this will slow down the development of resistance to the Bt toxin by various pests—particularly the corn-borer and pink boll-worm.

Unfortunately the refuge plans are "based in large part on computer models and not on large-scale field experiments . . . elements of the plans are highly controversial among entomologists and others who believe they are inadequate to forestall the evolution of resistant pests," says Rebecca Goldburg of Environmental Defense.[12]

Additionally, the new EPA rules have very weak enforcement provisions—requiring biotech seed companies to instruct farmers about the new rules and make sure they are complying. Biotech seed firms, not the EPA, are supposed to work with the farmers to report any adverse effects to Monarchs or other wildlife as a result of the genetically engineered crops.

WHO'S RESPONSIBLE FOR GENETIC CONTAMINATION?

THE THREAT of unknown genetically engineered pollen flying through the air to pollute another farmer's land is considered "one of the GM hot potatoes," according to Dr. Charles Benbrook[13] (see chapter 3 for more details). Already a major organic food company,

Terra Prima, lost hundreds of thousands of dollars when it discovered that the organic corn it was using was contaminated.[14]

But so far, neither the EPA or USDA are regulating problems associated with genetic drift, and there are no existing regulations to deal with it.

The states of Nebraska and Minnesota have introduced legislation that would establish liability for the manufacturers of the seed if genetic contamination or other environmental damage occurs. Similar legislation is expected to be introduced in the U.S. Congress in 2000.

WHY IS THERE NO LABELING OF GENETICALLY ENGINEERED FOODS?

IF THE U.S. had comprehensive labeling of genetically engineered foods this book would not have to be written. Despite nearly fifty different genetically engineered foods on the market, and overwhelming public support for labeling, the FDA has stuck by its 1992 decision not to label these radically new foods.

Yet the FDA does not seem to hesitate to require or allow numerous other types of labels for food. For example, labeling for kosher products, sugar, artificial flavoring, salt, cholesterol, preservatives are all allowed, and labels on orange and other juices must indicate whether they are from concentrate.

Yet, there is no labeling requirement for genetically engineered foods in the U.S. Under the Food Drug and Cosmetic Act, labeling is required when something is a "material fact" to consumers. The FDA has determined that in the case of genetically engineered foods, a "material fact" applies only when a food contains a known allergen, or decreases the nutritional value of the food.[15]

In objection to the FDA's labeling policy, the Center for Food Safety and the Alliance for Bio-Integrity filed a major lawsuit which brought together consumers, environmentalists, organic farmers, chefs, and religious leaders—all demanding that the FDA require labeling and safety testing of genetically engineered foods.

Members of the U.S. Congress are starting to respond to the growing call for labeling. In November 1999, a letter signed by a bi-partisan group of forty seven Members of Congress was sent to the Food and Drug Administration calling for the labeling of genetically engineered foods.

The signers of the letter, circulated by House Minority Whip David Bonior (D-MI), disagreed with the FDA's interpretation of the Federal Food, Drug, and Cosmetic Act, arguing that the Act was intended to ensure that consumers are provided thorough information and are not misled about the characteristics of their food. The members of Congress who signed the letter asserted that the FDA is required to label genetically engineered or modified foods under current law.

In the Meantime, Congressman Dennis Kucinich (D-OH) has introduced the Genetically Engineered Food Right to Know Act, which would require mandatory labeling of genetically engineered foods. Senator Barbara Boxer (D-CA) has introduced companion legislation on the Senate. The bills would also apply to animals fed genetically engineered material but would not require restaurants to comply with labeling. The label would read: "United States government notice: This product contains genetically engineered material, or was produced with a genetically engineered material."

The biotech and food industry have strongly opposed the Kucinich bill and all forms of mandatory labeling. The National Food Processors Association (NFPA) and the Alliance for Better Foods (funded by food trade associations) are pushing for so-called voluntary industry labeling. The NFPA also is suggesting additional information about genetically engineered food be provided through brochures, special displays, or toll-free numbers. As part of the FDA's new proposed rules, the agency has set up guidelines for voluntary labeling of genetically engineered, or non-genetically engineered foods. Of course, voluntary labeling products as "GE-free" places extra costs and burdens on companies that choose not to use the technology. Additionally, any voluntary labeling will be used sporadically within the food industry. It will be surprising if any food companies decide to label their products as "genetically engineered."

In March 2000, Representative Kucinich went a step further and introduced legislation that would completely revamp the FDA approval process for genetically engineered crops, requiring new crops to undergo the same type of rigorous safety testing that is required of new food additives.

GE BILLS AT THE STATE AND LOCAL LEVEL

WHILE REGULATORY activity has been slow to move forward at the federal level, it is hopping at the state level.

- In **California,** state legislators have introduced labeling legislation in the state Senate.
- In **Nebraska,** a state senator has introduced a bill that would hold makers of genetically modified seeds liable for damages if the plants cross-pollinate with a neighbor's crops.
- In **Vermont,** state legislators have introduced a bill which would place a one year moratorium on growing genetically engineered crops, while the effects of GE crops are studied further.
- In **Minnesota,** state legislators have introduced three separate bills. One would place a five-year moratorium on the planting of genetically engineered crops. The second would place liability of any environmental damage caused by engineered crops squarely on the seed companies—and not farmers. And the final bill is a strict mandatory labeling bill.
- In **Michigan**, a strict labeling bill has been introduced at the state legislature.
- In **West Virginia**, a bill was introduced that would make any food served in schools to be genetically-engineered free.

- In **Maryland**, lawmakers are considering legislation that would ban use of "Terminator" seeds in that state.
- In **New York** state, legislation has been introduced calling for a five-year moratorium on the planting of genetically engineered crops beginning in the year 2001.
- In **Berkeley**, the City Council passed a resolution calling for federal labeling of genetically engineered foods in December 1999.
- In **Boston**, the City Council called for a moratorium in March 2000 on genetically engineered foods and crops until further testing is done. The Council called for Federal labeling for those that have been approved.

WHAT SHOULD BE LABELED?

THERE IS little debate that whole food crops, such as genetically engineered corn or potatoes would be simple to label. But what about processed foods that contain ingredients made from genetically engineered plants such as canola oil, corn flour, cottonseed oil, or lecithin? And what percentage of genetically engineered material would trigger the need for a label?

Under the Kucinich bill, processed foods that contain .1 percent of genetically engineered material would have to be labeled as such. That is the lowest percentage at which foods can be reliably tested at the present time for genetically engineered material. Genetic ID, based in Iowa, was the world's first laboratory to offer GMO testing in 1996 and now licenses its DNA testing technique to laboratories around the world. DNA testing costs between $200–$400. But Monsanto's Roundup Ready soybeans can be detected with a simple $5.75 protein-based test being sold by Strategic Diagnostics Inc. (SDI), of Newark, Delaware., which produces results in three to five minutes—acting similar to a home pregnancy test. Early next year, SDI expects to offer tests that can identify four popular varieties of genetically engineered

Bt corn. (There are currently thirteen varieties of engineered corn on the market.) Maine-based EnviroLogix already makes a $3.50 quick test for Bt corn.

There are still technical difficulties involved in testing for some processed foods—including, for example, corn flakes. Highly processed sugars and oils also make it difficult to test because they have few proteins from which to extract DNA. The processing of products like corn syrup has helped serve as a cover for some food companies. For example, Coca-Cola tells consumers that it "does not use ingredients that are genetically modified."[16] But upon further questioning, the company argues that any genetically engineered ingredients they may use are destroyed in the processing. But Coca-Cola will not guarantee that the corn used in its corn syrup is genetically engineered free.

Nevertheless, the issue of what constitutes a genetically engineered product, and what should require labeling will likely be a hotly debated topic in the coming years.

WHAT FOOD PRODUCTS, INGREDIENTS, AND COMPANIES SHOULD YOU AVOID?

IF YOU want to avoid eating genetically engineered food, you will face several obstacles. The number-one hurdle is the lack of labeling. The absence of labeling muddles things at every step of the food chain. While a farmer knows whether his crops are genetically engineered, the companies that buy his harvest generally follow a "don't ask, don't tell" policy—although that may change soon. Until the point of purchase, genetically engineered crops and conventional crops are mixed together in giant grain elevators, as well as containers on trucks, train cars, barges, and ships—with possible contamination at each stage of the transportation chain. Food companies that buy the crops as ingredients for their products then buy the mixed crop, and use it to produce their food products. And when there is once again no labeling on the final package, you along with the rest of American consumers are pretty much left in the dark.

To become an informed food detective, you are going to have to learn how to read labels, know what genetically engineered foods are on the market, and understand what ingredients are likely to have been made from genetically engineered crops. It will take diligence. But, as we discuss in chapters 7 and 8, finding food that is not genetically engineered is not only possible—it can have great rewards.

The most common genetically engineered foods are also staples in many of our diets: corn, soy, canola, dairy products, and cottonseed oil, commonly used in vegetable oils. Thankfully, most of these genetically engineered foods are not in supermarkets in the form of whole foods, which are found in the produce section (although many of the foods in supermarket dairy cases come from cows injected with rBGH). In fact, most genetically engineered crops are used in animal feed or used as ingredients in processed foods—particularly corn, canola, and soy. It is estimated that at least 60 percent of processed foods on the market currently contain ingredients derived from genetically engineered soybeans alone.

In the ensuing pages, we will take you through some of the main genetically engineered foods and their derivative ingredients. Keep in mind that these ingredients will not be labeled as genetically engineered. However, because genetically engineered crops are intermingled with conventional crops, there is a good chance that they contain some genetically engineered material. The approach we outline in this book helps you identify foods that may be genetically engineered, and foods that you know are not. Armed with this information you should be able to dramatically decrease your consumption of genetically engineered foods and ingredients.

Canola (Rapeseed oil)

Chicory, red-hearted (Radicchio)

Corn—includes sweet corn and popcorn

Cotton

Flax

Papaya

Potato

Soybean

Squash

Sugarbeet

Tomato

Source: Union of Concerned Scientists[1]

GENETICALLY ENGINEERED FOODS AND DERIVATIVES

THE FIRST step is to simply commit to memory the crops listed, and know the numerous ingredients and derivatives that are commonly used in all kinds of processed foods that can find their way into your shopping cart.

Several large food companies, including Coca-Cola, have argued that ingredients made from genetically engineered crops should not constitute genetically engineered ingredients—or define their product as "genetically engineered." Coca-Cola claims that the DNA from any genetically engineered crops is destroyed during processing which creates oils, syrups, and other derivatives. However, there is evidence that this is not the case. According to Dr. Gordon Wiseman of RHM Technology in Buckinghamshire, U.K., a company that tests for genetically engineered content in food, all soy lecithin and up to 50 percent of oil samples contain enough DNA to still test positive as being genetically engineered after processing.[2]

Below is a list of "prime suspects" of foods that have been genetically engineered. We have listed the whole food, derivatives, and common products that may contain these ingredients. Much of this information has been gathered by the non-profit organization, Mothers for Natural Law[3]:

- **Soybeans**—*Derivatives: lecithin, soybean oil, soy flour, soy protein, soy isolates, genistein.* Lecithin E322 is the most common additive in food. Used as an emulsifier lecithin can be found in as much as 60 percent of all processed foods. Used in bread and bakery products, chocolate, margarine, cheese spread, mayonnaise, powdered milk and baby milk, cream, cheese spreads, fresh pasta, flans, mousses.[4] Products that may contain genetically engineered soy derivatives: vitamin E, tofu dogs, cereals, veggie burgers and sausages, tamari, soy sauce, chips, ice cream, frozen yogurt, infant formula, sauces, protein powder, margarine, soy cheeses, crackers, breads, cookies, chocolates, candies, fried foods, shampoo, bubble bath, cosmetics, enriched flours and pastas;

- **Corn**—*Derivatives: corn syrup, corn fructose, corn starch, corn dextrose, corn oil, corn flour.* Products that may contain genetically engineered corn derivatives: vitamin C, tofu dogs, chips, candies, ice cream, infant formula, salad dressings, tomato sauces, breads, cookies, cereals, baking powder, alcohol, vanilla, margarine, soy sauce, tamari, soda, fried foods, powdered sugar, enriched flours and pastas. There are several other food ingredients created from corn that are not easily identified as corn products. Those include the following:

  Dextrose, glucose, maltose, fructose, sucrose (syrups and solids)—Sugars processed from corn syrup used in sweet products like fruit and soft drinks.

  Maltodextrin—an industrial carbohydrate filler derived from corn. It's found in many processed foods such as gravy mixes and flavored chips—and used in cooked processed meats such as sliced ham and chicken, and in dry baby foods.[5]

Xanthan Gum (E415)—Derived from corn sugar, a thickener in ice cream, salad dressings and confectionery.

- **Canola**—*Derivatives: oil.* Products that may contain genetically engineered canola derivatives: chips, salad dressings, cookies, margarine, soaps, detergents, soy cheeses, fried foods.

- **Cotton**—*Derivatives: cottonseed oil, vegetable oil, cotton fabric.* Products that may contain genetically engineered cotton or its derivatives: clothes, linens, chips, peanut butter, crackers, cookies.

- **Potatoes**—*Derivatives: potato starch and flour.* The only genetically engineered potato variety is the Russet Burbank. Products that may contain genetically engineered potatoes or derivatives: unspecified processed or restaurant potato products (fries, mashed, baked, mixes, etc.), chips, Passover products, vegetable pies, soups.

- **Tomatoes**—No plum or roma tomatoes have been genetically engineered. But one variant of cherry tomato has, as have regular tomatoes. Products that may contain genetically engineered tomatoes or derivatives: sauces, purees, pizza, lasagna, and all processed Italian and Mexican foods.

- **Papaya**—Currently the only fruit genetically engineered. Others in development include: apples, grapes, strawberries, pineapples, bananas, melons.

- **Crook-Necked Yellow Squash**—Can be found in whole form, or in some baby foods.

- **Dairy Products**—Milk, cheese, butter, buttermilk, sour cream, yogurt, whey. Milk from cows injected with the recombinant Bovine Growth Hormone (rBGH) is mixed together with conventionally-produced milk, creating an identification problem similar to other genetically engineered crops. Find out more about genetically engineered-free dairy products in chapter 7. Cheese poses some unique problems. Several types of rennet are used for making cheese—including genetically engineered versions called chymosin or chymax, as well as animal rennet. The term "microbial enzyme" on a cheese package may refer to vegetable rennet (a natural enzyme from a mold), but this term is also used for genetically engineered rennet. "Vegetarian cheeses" may also contain genetically engineered rennet or vegetable rennet. According to the Consumers Union, some 60 percent of all hard cheese products in the U.S. are made with an engineered form of rennet.

SPECIFIC GENETICALLY ENGINEERED INGREDIENTS

ASIDE FROM genetically engineered whole foods, there are a number of specific ingredients that have been genetically engineered. The list below names the ingredient and some common products where it is used.[6]

- **Aspartame** (also known as NutraSweet)—a genetically engineered chemical that is usually found in diet soft drinks—but is also in over 9,000 products, including children's vitamins and medicines, chewing gum, many low-fat products, such as jelly, jam, and yogurt, and in some candy.
- **Baker's Yeast**—Genetically engineered yeast has been on the market for several years. It has been engineered to speed up the production of enzymes responsible for dough fermentation.
- **Brewer's Yeast**—Used primarily in beer, it has an enzyme that makes it produce more alcohol. It is unclear how frequently it is used.
- **Riboflavin** (Vitamin B2)—Engineered to increase the bac-

teria production of riboflavin and has an antibiotic resistance marker. It is used to fortify or enhance nutritionally many processed foods such as baby foods, breakfast cereals, fruit drinks, and vitamin-enriched milk—also in vitamin supplements.

- **Alpha Amylase**—An enzyme which breaks down starch—producing more sugars for the starch to work—used in cereals, soft drinks, beer and wine.
- **Hemicellulase**—Used to improve the strength of gluten in bread flour.
- **Lipase and Triaclyglycerol**—Genetically engineered enzyme used to break down fats—could be used in the manufacture of margarine, chocolate, and bakery goods.

FOODS TESTING POSITIVE

THERE HAS been no comprehensive testing of all food products on the market to find out which have genetically engineered ingredients—and which don't. However, there have been several random samplings of commonly found food products. The most recent sampling was done in September 1999 by the highly respected Consumers Union, publisher of *Consumer Reports.*[7] The *New York Times* and Greenpeace have also paid for similar testing.

Listed here are food products that have tested positive for genetically engineered ingredients based on sampling by the above three sources. Keep in mind that the food industry estimates that 60–75 percent of all processed foods in U.S. supermarkets likely contain genetically engineered ingredients:

- Alpo Dry Pet Food
- Aunt Jemima Pancake Mix
- Ball Park Franks
- Betty Crocker Bac-os Bacon Flavor Bits
- Boca Burger Chef Max's Favorite

- Bravos Tortilla Chips
- Duncan Hines Cake Mix
- Enfamil ProSobee Soy Formula
- Frito-Lay Fritos Corn Chips
- Gardenburger →
- General Mills Total Corn Flakes Cereal
- Green Giant Harvest Burgers
- Heinz 2 Baby Cereal
- Jiffy Corn Muffin Mix
- Kellogg's Corn Flakes
- Light Life Gimme Lean
- McDonald's McVeggie Burgers
- Morning Star Farms Better 'n Burgers →
- Nabisco Snackwell's Granola Bars
- Nestle Carnation Alsoy Infant Formula
- Old El Paso Taco Shells →
- Ovaltine Malt Powdered Beverage Mix
- Post Blueberry Morning Cereal
- Quaker Chewy Granola Bars
- Quaker White Cheddar Corn Cakes
- Quaker Yellow Corn Meal
- Quick Loaf Bread Mix
- Similac Isomil Soy Formula
- Ultra Slim Fast →

FOOD COMPANIES TESTING POSITIVE FOR GENETICALLY ENGINEERED INGREDIENTS:

MOST MAJOR U.S. food companies are using genetically engineered foods, ingredients or derivatives. If they haven't taken specific steps to source GE-free crops, then they are buying crops that have been genetically engineered.

As you will read in chapter 7, a growing number of companies are going GE-free. This means that their entire brand-name product line is free of genetically engineered ingredients. Below is a list of food companies whose products have tested positive for genetically engineered ingredients. Food companies buy ingredients in bulk. If one product is found to contain genetically engineered ingredients, it is likely that those same ingredients are being used in the company's other products.

- Crisco (shortening)
- Frito, Dorito, Tostito (corn chips)
- ~~Green Giant~~ (harvest burger)
- Isomil and ProSobee (soy formula)
- Kellogg's (corn flakes)
- ~~Kraft~~ (salad dressings)
- McDonald's (french fries)
- Nabisco (sundry)
- Nestle (chocolate, dairy)
- Old El Paso (taco shells)
- Ovaltine (malt beverage)
- Parkay (margarine)
- Pillsbury (sundry)
- Procter & Gamble (sundry)
- Quaker Mills (sundry)
- Wesson (vegetable oils)

Source: Consumer Reports, September 1999, NYT, 9–8–99.

GE-FREE IN OTHER COUNTRIES, BUT NOT IN THE UNITED STATES

Thus far, no major U.S. food companies have decided to not use genetically engineered ingredients in all their products, although some have taken small steps forward. This is frustrating for many U.S. consumers because many of these same companies have pledged to go GE-free in Europe.

Here are a list of some of the food companies that have gone GE-free in some countries or all of Europe, but have not done so in the U.S.:

- Coca-Cola
- General Mills
- Heinz
- Hershey's
- Kellogg's
- Kraft
- McDonald's
- Burger King
- Nabisco
- Nestle
- PepsiCo
- Pillsbury
- Procter & Gamble
- Quaker Oats
- Safeway
- Tengelmann (majority owner of A&P Supermarkets)

THE TWENTY-FIVE LARGEST
U.S. FOOD COMPANIES

NEARLY ALL of the largest food companies in the U.S. have refused to take steps to confirm that they are not using genetically engineered foods. In fact, the top 100 U.S. food companies all appear to be using genetically engineered ingredients in their foods. The environmental organization Friends of the Earth has contacted all of the top 100 companies and asked whether they are using genetically engineered ingredients. Most of the 100 have refused to comment.

Here is a list of the top twenty-five U.S. food companies, their contact information, and primary food products.[8] While not all of the companies responded to our requests for their position on genetically engineered foods, many did. Coca-Cola argued that any genetically engineered ingredients they may be using are destroyed in the processing. Frito-Lay pointed out that 95 percent of the corn they use is GE-free, but could not vouch for the rest of their ingredients. And Dole states that none of the fruit and vegetables they use are genetically engineered, however, it does not label its products GE-free, and doesn't confirm that other ingredients such as sweeteners are GE-free. We've listed abbreviated versions of company statements below. Please keep in mind that corporate leaders change jobs and policies all the time. We have made every effort to ensure that the information below is correct at the present time. We encourage you to contact the company directly for their latest position on GE foods.

1. **Philip Morris Companies, Inc.** (owner of Kraft Foods)
    Betsy Holden, President & CEO
    3 Lakes Dr.
    Northfield, IL 60093
    Phone: 847-646-2000
    Fax: 847-646-2922
    Web sites: www.philipmorris.com, www.kraftfoods.com
    BRANDS: Kool-Aid, Maxwell House Coffee, Di Giorno, Stove Top, Oven Classics, Toblerone, Country Time Lemonade, Cheez-Whiz, Jell-O, Kraft Mayonnaise, Miracle Whip, Post Cereals

2. **ConAgra Inc.**
    Bruce Rohde, Chairman & CEO
    One Con Agra Drive,
    Omaha, NE 61802-5001
    Phone: 402-595-4000 (General), 1-800-323-9985 (Healthy Choice Consumer Line)
    Web site: www.conagra.com
    BRANDS: Montfort, La Choy, Swiss Miss, Healthy Choice, Hunts, Butterball, Orville Redenbacher's, Eckrich, Wesson

3. **PepsiCo Inc.** (owner of Frito-Lay)
    Roger A. Enrico, Chairman & CEO
    700 Anderson Hill Road

Purchase, NY 10577
Phone: 914-253-2000
Fax: 914-253-2070
Web site: www.pepsico.com

BRANDS: Pepsi, Frito-Lay, Tropicana & PBG, Chee-tos, Grandma's Cookies, Sun Chips, Aquafina, Alegro

Frito-Lay (owned by Pepsico)
Steven S. Reinemund, CEO
7701 Legacy Drive
Plano, TX 75024
Phone: 972-334-7000
Web site: www.fritolay.com

BRANDS: Cheetos Cheese Flavored Snacks, Cracker Jack, Doritos Tortilla Chips, Fritos Corn Chips, Funyuns, Onion Flavored Rings, Grandmas Cookies

COMPANY STATEMENT: "Now that there is a renewed interest in biotechnology and some consumer confusion exists, we did not feel it appropriate to ask our growers to include Bt crops in what they sell us. At the same time, we have no plans to market or advertise any claim of 'Genetically Modified-Free' products . . . Since we are also a large buyer of agricultural commodities, and more than a quarter of the North American crop is derived from biotechnology, just like other food companies, we could have biotechnology ingredients in our products."

4. Coca-Cola Enterprises Inc.

Douglas Ivestor, Chairman & CEO
P.O. Box 723040
Atlanta, GA 31139
Phone: 770-989-3000
Fax: 770-989-3640
Web site: www.cocacola.com

BRANDS: Coke, Fanta, Fruitopia, Minute Maid, Nestea, Powerade

COMPANY STATEMENT: "The Coca-Cola Company does not use ingredients that are genetically modified." When asked for further clarification, a consumer affairs specialist said that any genetically engineered ingredients that the company might use are destroyed in the processing.

5. Mars Inc.

Forrest E. Mars Jr., President & CEO
6885 Elm Street
McLean, VA 22101
Phone: 703-821-4900
Fax: 703-448-9678
Web site: www.mars.com
BRANDS: M&M, Snickers, Dove, Milky Way, Twix, Starburst, Mars, Skittles, Uncle Ben's, Kal Kan, Pedigree Dog Food

6. IBP Inc.

Robert Peterson, Chairman & CEO
26999 Central Park Blvd.
Suite 300
Southfield, MI 48076
Phone: 1-800-347-7675
Web site: www.lbpinc.com
BRANDS: American Favorite, Butcher Boy, Fred's IBP, Supreme Lean, Wilson's Food Service, Wilson's Continental Deli, Thorn Apple Valley

7. Sara Lee Corp.

John Bryan, Chairman & CEO
3 First National Plaza
Chicago, IL 60602
Phone: 312-274-8200, 1-800-323-7117 (customer service)
Fax: 312-274-8829
Web site: www.saralee.com
BRANDS: Ball Park, Hillshire Farm, Jimmy Dean, Sara Lee

8. H. J. Heinz Company

William Johnson, President & CEO
600 Grant St.
Pittsburgh, PA 15219
Phone: 412-456-5700, 1-800-872-2229 (Heinz Baby Food Consumer Relations)
Fax: 412-456-6128
Web site: www.heinz.com
BRANDS: Budget Gourmet, Heinz, Ore-Ida, Starkist, Weight Watchers, Heinz baby food, Heinz Ketchup
COMPANY STATEMENT: "Heinz has responded to concerns about GMOs throughout the world and will continue to be responsive to changes in consumer expectations as well as regulatory policy. We seek to avoid ingredients from GM sources. For example, in the case of tomatoes, we only use tomatoes bred utilizing traditional breeding technology. Additionally, we are working with non-tomato ingredient suppliers to understand the source of these ingredients and the future of the supply."

9. Nabisco Holdings Corp

James M. Kilts, President & CEO
7 Campus Dr.
Parsippany, NJ 07054
Phone: 973-682-5000, 1-800-932-7800 (products)
Fax: 973-503-2202 (products)
Web site: www.nabisco.com
BRANDS: Oreo, Chips Ahoy!, Fig Newtons, Ritz, A1 Steak Sauce, Grey Poupon, Planters, LifeSavers, Bubble Yum, Del Monte, Red Oval Farm, Snack Well's, Stella D'Oro, WheatThins, Triscuts, Oat Thins, Mystic, Honey Maid, Planters, Ritz, Now + Later, Better Cheddars

10. Bestfoods

Merrill E. Eastman, CEO

International Plaza
700 Sylvan Avenue
Englewood Cliffs, NJ 07632
Phone: 201-894-4000, 1-800-338-8831, 1-800-356-3314
(consumer lines)
Fax: 210-894-2950, attn: Irene McCall
Web site: www.bestfoods.com
BRANDS: Hellmann's, Karo, Knorr, Mazola, Mueller's,
   Skippy, Boboli, Entenmann's, Thomas'
COMPANY STATEMENT: "Bestfoods uses only approved
   ingredients conforming to health, safety, and quality
   assurance standards set by the U.S. government and
   other governmental bodies worldwide. These ingredients include some that may have been derived from
   genetically-modified corn, soybean and canola."

11. Nestle

Joe Weller, Chairman & CEO
800 North Brand Blvd.
Glendale, CA 91203
Phone: 818-549-6000, 1-800-452-1971 (consumer line)
Fax: 818-549-6952
Web site: www.nestleusa.com, www.verybestbaking.com,
www.verybestbaby.com.
BRANDS: Carnation, Nestle Candy, Coffee Mate, Juicy
   Juice, Stouffer's, Taster's Choice, Nestle Quick, Nestle
   Carnation Baby Formula, Butterfinger, Ortega
COMPANY STATEMENT: "In countries where public opinion
   rejects ingredients derived from genetically modified
   crops, even though food legislation permits their use,
   Nestle respects the consumers' preferences and will
   provide its customers, in as far technically possible,
   with products that do not contain these ingredients.
   Nestle will continue to use ingredients derived from
   genetically modified crops where we have complete

confidence in their safety and where they are generally accepted by consumers."

12. Tyson Foods
Wayne Britt, CEO
2210 W. Oaklawn Drive
Springdale, AR 72762
Phone: 501-290-4000, 1-800-243-6332 (consumer affairs)
Web site: www.tyson.com
BRANDS: Arctic Ice, Cooking Made Easy, Holly Farms, Tastybird, Tyson, Weaver, Louis Kemp, Quick-to-Fix

13. Kellogg Company
Carlos M. Gutierrez, CEO
One Kellogg Square, P.O. Box 3599
Battle Creek, MI 49016
Phone: 616-961-2000, 1-800-962-1413 (consumer affairs)
Fax: 616-961-2871
Web site: www.kelloggs.com
BRANDS: Apple Jacks, Cocoa Krispies, Corn Flakes, Crackel'n Oat Bran, Special K, Raisin Bran, Just Right, Rice Krispies, PopTarts, Lender's Bagels, Eggo
COMPANY STATEMENT: "Kellogg Company uses grain from a number of suppliers in our country, so our supply would likely include biotechnology-produced grain in the same proportion that it occurs in the United States supply."

14. Campbell Soup Company
David Johnson, President & CEO
Campbell Place
Camden, NJ 08103
Phone: 856-342-4800 (1-800-257-8443)
Fax: 856-342-3878
Web site: www.campbellsoup.com

BRANDS: 75 percent of U.S. soup market, Franco-American, Godiva, Hungry-Man, Pace, Pepperidge Farm, Prego, SpaghettiOs, V8

COMPANY STATEMENT: "Campbell's use of genetically engineered ingredients is small, restricted primarily to part of its supply of products derived from corn and soybeans."

15. General Mills

Stephen Sanger, CEO
Number One General Mills Blvd.
Minneapolis, MN 55440
Phone: 612-540-2311, 1-800-328-1144 (consumer line)
Web site: www.generalmills.com

Brands: Bisquick, Bugles, Fruit Roll-Ups, Gold Medal, Betty Crocker, Nature Valley, Yoplait, Colombo, Pop Secret, Bac-Os, Golden Grahams, Cheerios, Cocoa Puffs, Chex, Fiber One, Total, Cinnamon Toast Crunch, Wheaties, Oatmeal Crisp, Pop-Secret, Raisin Nut Bran, Trix

COMPANY STATEMENT: "Because of the growing use of biotechnology by farmers and the way that grain gets commingled in storage and shipment, it's certainly possible that some of our products may contain ingredients that have been improved through biotechnology."

16. Pillsbury Co.

John N. Lilly, President & CEO
200 S. Sixth Street
Minneapolis, MN 55402
Phone: 612-330-4966, 1-800-767-4466
Web site: www.pillsbury.com

BRANDS: Green Giant, Häagen-Däzs, Hungry Jack, Old El Paso, Pillsbury, Progresso

17. Quaker Oats Co.

Robert Morrison, Chairman, President & CEO

Quaker Tower 321 N. Clark St.
Chicago, IL 60610
Phone: 312-222-7111
Consumer Affairs
P.O. Box 049003
Chicago, IL 60604-9003
Phone: 1-800-367-6287 (Consumer Line for Old-Fashioned and Quick Quaker Oats)
1-800-407-2247 (Consumer Line for Aunt Jemina)
Web site: www.quakeroats.com

BRANDS: Aunt Jemima, Cap'n Crunch, Life, Golden Grain, Gatorade, Noodle-Roni, Quaker Rice & Popcorn Cakes, Rice-A-Roni

COMPANY STATEMENT: "While Quaker does not require or exclude the use of these [GE] foods, the use of corn, canola and soya developed through food biotechnology is widespread. Currently, there is no system in place in the United States that separates these foods. So, there is a high probability that some of Quaker's products contain foods developed through biotechnology."

18. Dole Food Co. Inc.

David Murdock, Chairman & CEO
P.O. Box 5132
Westlake Village, CA 91359-5132
Phone: 818-879-6600, 1-800-232-8888 (consumer center)
Fax: 818-879-4893
Web site: www.dole.com

BRANDS: Classic Salad, Complete Salad, Fruit Bowls, Lunch for One, Special Blends

COMPANY STATEMENT: "ALL of the Dole brand fruit and vegetables, whether grown by Dole, or by individual farmers who grow specially for Dole, are the same fruit and vegetable natural varieties that have always been available and that Dole has always provided to its consumers. *None* of these fruit and vegetable varieties sold under the Dole brand trace their origin to new scientific research techniques popularly referred to as 'genetic engineering.'"

19. Hershey Foods Corp.

Kenneth Wolfe, Chairman & CEO
100 Crystal A. Drive
Hershey, PA 17033
Phone: 717-534-4200, 1-800-468-1714 (Consumer Relations)
Web site: www.hersheys.com
BRANDS: chocolate confectionary, non chocolate confectionary, chips, drinks, ice-cream toppings, Almond Joy, 5th Avenue, Cadbury's Candies, Caramellos, Chocolate Chips, Good + Plenty, Heath Bar, Hershey's Jolly Rancher, Kisses, KitKat, Milk Duds, Reese's, Oh Henry, Whoppers

20. Procter & Gamble Company

A. G. Lafley, President & CEO
One Procter & Gamble Plaza
Cincinnati, OH 45202
Phone: 513-983-1100, 1-800-331-3774 (consumer line)
Web site: www.pg.com
BRANDS: Pringles, Crisco, Jif, Millstone, Olean, Folgers, Sunny Delight, Hawaiian Punch

21. Smithfield Foods Inc.

Joseph W. Luter III, Chairman & CEO
200 Commerce Street
Smithfield, VA 23430
Phone: 757-365-3000, 757-357-4321 (packing plant)
Web site: 757-365-3017
Web site: www.smithfieldfoods.com
BRANDS: Gwaltney, Lykes, Smithfield Premium, Peyton's, Jamestown

22. Flowers Industries

Amos R. McMullian, Chairman & CEO
1919 Flowers Circle
Thomasville, GA 31757
Phone: 912-226-9110, 912-226-9116 (Flowers Bakeries)
Web site: www.flowersindustries.com
BRANDS: Keebler, Cheez-It, Famous Amos, Hydrox, Mrs. Smith's, Nature's Own, Sunshine, Vienna Fingers

23. Hormel Foods Corp.

Joel Johnson, Chairman, President & CEO
One Hormel Place
Austin, MN 55912
Phone: 507-437-5611, 1-800-523-4635 (Consumer Affairs)
Fax: 507-437-5129 (Administration), 507-437-9852 (consumer affairs)
Web site: www.hormel.com
BRANDS: Fast 'N Easy, Homeland, Light Lean, Little Sizzlers, Old Smokehouse, Sandwich Maker, Wranglers, Dinty Moore, Chi-Chi's, Jennie-O, El Torito
COMPANY STATEMENT: ". . . there have been a variety of developments in plant genetics that have significantly improved crop productivity and food quality . . . innovation and advancements in technology are a very important part of our mission and our responsibility to you as a valued customer. Hormel Foods will, therefore, continue to support the crop and vegetable industries' efforts to provide the safest and highest quality products available."

24. Suiza Foods Corp.

Gregg L. Engles, Chairman & CEO
2515 McKinney Ave., Ste. 1200, Lock Box 30
Dallas, TX 75201
Phone: 214-303-3400
Fax: 214-303-3499

Web site: www.suizafoods.com

25. Dean Foods
Howard Dean, Chairman & CEO
3600 N. River Road
Franklin Park, IL 60131
Phone: 847-678-1680
Fax: 847-233-5508 (Investor Relations)
Corporate Dairy Division
Eric Blanchard, President Dairy Division
O'Hare International Center II
10255 W. Higgins Rd.
Rosemont, IL 60018
Phone: 847-699-8310, 1-800-395-7004 (milk consumer response line)
Web site: www.deanfoods.com
BRANDS: Berkeley Farms, Carnation Coffee Mate Liquid, Dairy Ease, Hillside, Meadow Brook, VeriFine

BABY FOODS AND HOSPITAL FEEDING

THE ONLY analysis done in the U.S. on baby food and hospital/nursing home food was commissioned by Greenpeace in 1999.[9] The findings revealed the presence of transgenic DNA from genetically engineered foods in several popular brands of baby foods and in nutritional supplements used for tube feeding in hospitals and nursing homes.

Gerber Mixed Cereal for Baby, a dry three-grain cereal mix for infants, tested positive for DNA from transgenic insect-resistant "Bt" corn and herbicide-tolerant "Roundup Ready" (RR) soybeans. Shortly after the findings of the study were announced, Gerber announced that it will go GE-free and substitute organic ingredients for its baby food. Heinz also announced that its baby would be GE-free. Additionally, while Enfamil, the baby for company, has announced that it is going GE-free, Nestle and Ross Nutrition (maker of Similac) will continue to use genetically engineered ingredients.

The two nutritional supplements produced by Novartis' IsoSource and Ross Products' Osmolite both contained transgenic DNA from RR soy.

VITAMINS AND SUPPLEMENTS

GENETICALLY ENGINEERED ingredients have found their way into supplements. Many of the source materials used to produce the most common vitamins are food commodities such as soy and corn. The proteins of the soy or corn remain intact throughout the vitamin making process. For instance, vitamin C is made with corn fructose—which may be genetically altered.

Because of these concerns, the National Nutritional Foods Association (NNFA), which represents retailers and manufacturers of dietary supplements, natural foods, and other products, recently filed a citizen petition with the FDA, demanding that the agency strengthen its evaluation process of genetically engineered foods and calling for more rigorous oversight of the new products. The NNFA wants to help manufacturers and consumers know more about genetically engineered ingredients in supplements.

RESTAURANTS

CONSUMERS ARE particularly vulnerable when it comes to genetically engineered foods in many restaurants. Restaurants are not required to label their food, and many chefs may not know whether their ingredients are genetically engineered or not. Most major fast food restaurants such as McDonald's and Burger King have told customers in Europe that they do not use genetically engineered ingredients. While no chain restaurants have made the same claim in the U.S., there is second-hand evidence that McDonald's, Burger King and Wendy's have requested that their potatoes used for fries not be genetically-engineered. (Find out more about efforts by chefs to go GE-free in chapter 7.) The *Wall Street Journal* reported in late April 2000 that McDonald's, Burger King, Frito-Lay, and Procter and Gamble have told their potato suppliers that they do not want genetically engineered potatoes.[10] Thus far, none of the fast food chains are labeling their potatoes as GE-free—perhaps hoping to not draw attention to other genetically engineered ingredients such as canola and soy. As listed earlier in this chapter, McDonald's veggie burger has already tested positive for containing genetically engineered ingredients—most likely soy. Also supporting the contention that the big three fast food chains are using GE-free potatoes was the statement by the Canadian company McCain's, the largest supplier of potatoes for french fries to fast food chains, that it would not use genetically engineered potatoes.[11]

WHICH COMPANIES AND STORES ARE GOING GE-FREE?

IN EUROPE, almost every major food manufacturer and supermarket chain has banned genetically engineered ingredients from its brand-name products (see chapter 5 for a country-by-country overview). This means that they will not sell genetically engineered foods, or ingredients derived from genetically engineered crops. Up until now, other than organic companies, very few U.S. food companies or supermarkets have banned the use of genetically engineered foods or ingredients for their brand name products.

Several supermarket chains, including Safeway and Albertsons, have banned genetically engineered foods in their European stores, but have decided not to do so in the U.S. According to Safeway in an October 22, 1999 letter to the Friends of the Earth, "We do not currently envision refraining from using GM (genetically modified) substances in our private label products or from selling GM foods."

But leaders of a new wave of popular, natural and organic food stores have taken a stand. In December 1999, Whole Foods and Wild Oats, the two largest natural food supermarket chains in the country, announced that they would ban the use of genetically engineered ingredients in their own brand-name food products and would pressure their suppliers to eliminate gene-altered ingredients from their product lines. Wild Oats will ultimately label their food as GE-free. This does not mean that all food products in these stores will not include genetically engineered ingredients—only that their store brands do not. Whole Foods has more than 600 products carrying its brand name. Wild Oats has about 700 products under its own brand.

"It's really not my position to say genetically engineered is a good thing or a bad thing," said Jim Lee, president and chief operating officer of Wild Oats. "It's a matter of having a shopping choice. A high percentage of our customers are opposed to anything artificially introduced into their food."[1]

Be on the look out for similar policies to be adopted at other major supermarket chains as consumer awareness about genetically engineered foods grows.

WHAT ABOUT FOOD COMPANIES?

While most major traditional U.S. supermarkets have been slow to act, several food companies have made certain specific products GE-free.

- Both Heinz's Earth's Best line, and Gerber—two of the biggest baby food makers—announced in 1999 that they would try to make their products genetically engineered-free, and Gerber went a step further declaring that it would substitute corn flour and soy flour that is "organic." The Gerber decision, in response to a letter from Greenpeace, was particularly important, given that the company is the largest baby food manufacturer in the country as well as being a subsidiary of Novartis—the giant Swiss-based biotech company.[2]

- In March 2000, Mead Johnson Nutritionals, maker of Enfamil baby formula, announced that it would go GE-free. Enfamil is one of the nation's largest producers of baby formulas. Prior to this announcement it was impossible to get GE-free baby formula in the U.S.
- Perhaps the most significant food company to go at least partially GE-free is Frito-Lay (owned by Pepsico), which in February 2000 announced that it had told its farmers not to grow genetically engineered corn. In 1999, Frito-Lay bought 1.2 billion pounds of corn to be used in products such as Doritos, Fritos, and Tostitos chips. More than 95 percent of the corn purchased by Frito-Lay comes from farmers that are under direct contract to the company.

It is unclear, however, how the company will take steps to guarantee that the other 5 percent of its corn is non-genetically engineered. In addition, Frito-Lay does buy some ingredients in bulk, including cooking oils, that could derive from genetically engineered crops. The company is not guaranteeing that its products are GE free, and Frito-Lay has stated that it currently has no plans to start marketing its products as GE free.

- In late April, the *Wall Street Journal* uncovered what had been rumored for many months, that several major food companies were asking for non-genetically engineered potatoes. J.R. Simplot Co., a major supplier of french fries to McDonald's, is instructing its farmers to stop growing genetically engineered Bt potatoes. JR Simplot was told not to grow the GE spuds by several companies including McDonald's, Burger King, Frito-Lay, and Procter and Gamble. "Virtually all the [fast food] chains have told us they prefer to take nongenetically modified potatoes," Fred Zerza, spokesman for closely held J.R. Simplot, told the *Journal*.[3]

- In October 1999, Hain Food Group Inc. announced that it would switch the oil it uses in its fryers from corn to safflower, and place labels on its Little Bear line of natural snacks, indicating that it contained no genetically engineered ingredients. Hain will use a "Pure Food" symbol to signify that the product contains no genetically engineered ingredients. Bearitos Tortilla Chips is the first Hain product with this label.[4]
- Worthington Foods Inc., which makes Morningstar Farms veggie burgers, announced in late 1999 that it would take genetically engineered soybeans out of its product.[5]
- Seagrams, one of the world's largest distillers, is telling farmers that it will not purchase genetically engineered corn.[6]

Other major natural and organic food companies that have made public statements indicating that they have gone GE-free include:

- Annie's Naturals
- Barbara's Bakery
- Eden's
- Lightlife Foods
- GeniSoy
- White Wave
- Northern Soy
- Walnut Acres
- Newman's Own
- SunRich
- Guiltless Gourmet
- Nature's Path
- Organic Valley
- Vitasoy
- Kettle Foods
- Pacific Grain and Foods

Source: Company Correspondence, People's Earth Network

COMPANIES BY TYPE OF PRODUCT

Below is a list of companies that have stated that they do not use genetically engineered ingredients. This list, largely put together by the non-profit Mothers for Natural Law, can be easily searched by food product.

- Flours—Arrowhead Mills; Eden flours.
- Sweeteners—Eden Organic Malted Grain Sweeteners, Kogee Organic Cane Sugar, Organic Cane Sugar, Pure USA Hone, Sucanat North America.
- Syrups—Eden Organic Malted Grain Sweeteners, Wholesome Foods Organic Backstrap Molasses, Andersons Pure Maple Syrup, Cary's Maple Syrup (premium), Hauke Honey Pure Maple Syrup, Spring Tree Pure Maple Syrup.
- Olive Oils (extra virgin)—Alessi Olio, Da Vinci, Eden Selected, Filippo Berio, Gourmet Aritrian, Grey Poupon, L'estronell, Odd Monk, Olitalia, Peloponnese, Spectrum Natural, Tassos.
- Other Oils—Eden (organic sesame, toasted sesame, hot pepper toasted sesame, and safflower oils), Sigg Grapeseed Oil, Olitalia Grapeseed Oil, Loriva Sesame Oil, Spectrum Natural (almond oil, apricot kernel oil, avocado oil, coconut oil, safflower oil, walnut oil).
- Vinegars—Da Vinci Balsamic, Eden Apple Cider, L'estronell River Run Hot Pepper, Spectrum Organic (raspberry wine, red wine, white wine).
- Salad Dressings and Condiments—Cross and Blackwell Capers, Spectrum Zesty Italian Dressing, Jaffa Gold Lemon Juice, Melinda Extra Hot Sauce, Annie's Farmhouse Maple Mustard, Earth Fire Products Chutney, Eden Organic Mustard (and imported condiments), Sandhill Mustard, Santa Barbara Olive Company California Ripe Large or Jumbo Pitted Olives, Muir Glen Organic Tomato Ketchup,

Cascadian Farm Organic Sauerkraut, Eden Organic Sauerkraut, Krinos Imported Grape Leaves.

- Nut and Fruit Butters—Arrowhead Mills (certified organic peanut butter, sesame tahini), Eastwind Nut Butters (peanut, cashew, tahini, almond), Eden Organic Apple Butter, Joyva Sesame Tahini, Maranata Roasted (pistachio butter, filbert butter, sunflower butter, almond butter), Maranata (sesame tahini, cashew butter, almond butter) Once Again Hazelnut Butter, Sahadi Sesame Butter, Santa Cruz Organic (apple apricot sauce, apple sauce), Westbrae Natural (raw sesame tahini, toasted tahini).

- Breads—French Meadow Bakery, Garden of Eatin (blue corn and corn tortillas), Lundberg Rice Cakes, Manna, New Pioneer Co-op (farm bread, olive farm, raisin pecan, sourdough, wheat).

- Canned Beans—American Prairie, Bearitos Refried Fat Free, Eden, Shari's, Westbrae Natural Garbanzo.

- Salsas—Garden Valley Naturals, Muir Glen, New Bounty Organic, Parrot.

- Pasta Sauces—Eden (spaghetti sauce, pizza-pasta sauce), Garden Valley Organic, Millina's Finest Organic, Muir Glen Organic.

- Pastas/Noodles—Eden, Millina's Finest, Vita Spelt.

- Tofu/Tempeh/Soy/Miso—American Pride Tofu, Earth Fire Products, Eden products, White Wave (organic wild rice tempeh, five grain tempeh, soy tempeh, sea veggie tempeh, organic tofu).

- Frozen Foods—Cascadian Farms (organic broccoli, corn, plain vegetables, raspberries, blueberries, strawberries), Sno-Pac (organic vegetables).

- Teas—Alvita, Celestial Seasonings (except for its vitamin enriched teas), Choice Organic, Eden Great Eastern Sun, Long Life Organic, Maharishi Ayur-Veda (Vata, Pitta and Kapha Churnas and Teas, and Raja's Cup), Traditional Medicinals, Yogi Organic.

- Juices—Organic with no vitamins added: After the Fall (Vermont Harvest Moon, apple cider, grape juice), Crofters (guava, strawberry, papaya, raspberry, apricot, pink lemonade), Eden (organic apple, organic tomato, organic cherry), Kedem (100 percent pure grape juice), Knudsen (cherry, grape, mango, pea, strawberry), Mountain Sun (organic strawberry, peach, blueberry, cranberry), Santa Cruz (ginger, apricot, cherry, raspberry, apple).
- Chips/snacks/candies—Eden, Little Bear Lite Organic Popcorn, Manischewitz Passover Matzos (tea matzos and whole wheat tea matzos), Reeds Crystallized Ginger, St. Claire Organic (winter mints, licorice sweets, cinnamon snaps, cherry sweets, lemon tarts, peppermints, cocoa sweets, ginger snaps), dried non-GE fruit (either unsweetened or approved non-GE sweetener), Westbrae Organic Potato Chips.

SEED COMPANIES

The Council for Responsible Genetics and High Mowing Organic Seed Farm have started a project called the Safe Seed Initiative. The effort asks seed companies to sign a pledge not to use genetically engineered seeds. Below is a list of companies that have explicitly agreed not to use genetically engineered seeds. (See page 190 for a complete list of organic seed companies, some of which have signed this pledge. Even those who haven't are likely to be GE-free.)

California:
Abundant Life Seed Foundation
PO Box 772
Port Townsend, WA 98368

Bountiful Gardens
   18001 Shafer Ranch Rd
   Willits, CA 95490

Environmental Seed Producers
   PO Box 2709
   Lompoc, CA 93438

Horse Creek Seed Santuary
   PO Box 1476
   Santa Cruz, CA 95061

KUSA Seed Research Foundation
   PO Box 761
   Ojai, CA 93024

Santa Barbara Heirloom Nursery
   PO Box 4235
   Santa Barbara, CA 93140

Colorado:
Beauty Beyond Belief Wildflower Seeds
   1730 So. College Ave, #104
   Fort Collins, CO 80525

Sunnyland Seeds
   PO Box 385
   Paradox, CO 81429

Connecticut:
New England Seed Co.
   3580 Main St, Bldg 10
   Hartford, CT 06120

Butterbrooke Farm
78 Barry Rd
Oxford, CT 06478

Florida:
The Pepper Gal
PO Box 23006
Ft. Lauderdale, FL 33307

Glendale Enterprises
297 Railroad Ave
De Funiak Springs, FL 32433

Florida Mycology Research Center
PO Box 18105
Pensacola, FL 32523

Idaho:
Seeds Trust & High Altitude Gardens
Bill McDorman
PO Box 1048
Hailey, ID 83333

Illinois:
Underwood Gardens
4N381 Maple Ave
Bensenville, IL 60106

Borries Open Pollinated Seed Corn Farm
16293 E. 1400th Ave
Teutopolis, IL 62567

Iowa:

Seed Savers Exchange
   3076 North Winn Rd
   Decorah, IA 52101

Sand Hill Preservation Center
   1878 230th St
   Calamus, IA 52729

Maine:

FedCo Seeds
   PO Box 520
   Waterville, ME 04903

Johnny's Selected Seeds
   310 Foss Hill Rd, Box 2580
   Albion, ME 04910

Maine Seed Saving Network
   PO Box 126
   Penobscot, ME 04476

Wood Prairie Farm
   49 Kinney Rd
   Bridgewater, ME 04735

Massachusetts:

Pioneer Valley Seed Savers
   888 Shelburne Falls Rd
   Conway, MA 01341

Missouri:

Baker Creek Heirloom Seeds
   2278 Baker Creek Rd
   Mansfield, MO 65704

Barney's Ginseng Patch
   433 SSE Highway B
   Montgomery City, MO 63361

Morgan County Wholesale
   Route 2, Box 35A
   Barnett, MO 65011

Montana:
Garden City Seeds
   778 Hwy. 93 N
   Hamilton, MT 59840

New Mexico:
Seeds of Change
   PO Box 15700
   Santa Fe, NM 87506

Deep Diversity
   PO Box 15700
   Santa Fe, NM 87506

North Carolina:
Boone's Native Seed Company
   PO Box 10363
   Raleigh, NC 27605

Christopher Weeks Peppers
   PO Box 3207
   Kill Devil Hills, NC 27948

Ohio:
Mellinger's Inc.
   2310 W. South Range Rd
   North Lima, OH 44452

Oregon:
Nichol's Garden Nursery
   1190 N. Pacific Hwy
   Albany, OR 97321

Peters Seed & Research
   PO Box 1472
   Myrtle Creek, OR 97457

Territorial Seed Company
   PO Box 157
   Cottage Grove, OR 97424

Horizon Herbs
   PO Box 69
   Williams, OR 97544

Wild Garden Seed
   PO Box 1509
   Philomath, OR 97370

Pennsylvania:
Heirloom Seeds
   PO Box 245
   West Elizabeth, PA 15088

Pepper Joe's
   1650 Pembroke Rd
   Norristown, PA 19403

Bethlehem Seed Company
   PO Box 1351
   Bethlehem, PA 18018

Heirloom Seed Project
  Landis Valley Museum
  2451 Kissel Hill Rd
  Lancaster, PA 17601

South Carolina:
Seeds for the South
  410 Whaley Pond Rd
  Graniteville, SC 29829

Vermont:
Arethusa Seed Farm
  PO Box 183
  Bakersfield, VT 05441

High Mowing Organic Seed Farm
  813 Brook Rd
  Wolcott, VT 05680

The Cook's Garden
  PO Box 535
  Londonderry, VT 05148

Zwaan Seeds
  PO Box 179
  Grafton, VT 05146

Ladybug Herbs of Vermont
  RR1 Box 3380
  Wolcott, VT 05680

Virginia:
Garden Medicinals & Culinaries
  PO Box 170
  Earlysville, VA 22936

Thomas Jefferson Center for Historic Plants
    PO Box 316
    Charlottesville, VA 22902

Washington:
Filaree Farm
    182 Conconully Hwy
    Okanogan, WA 98840

Fungi Perfecti
    PO Box 7634
    Olympia, WA 98507

Canada:
Richters Herbs
    357 Hwy 47
    Goodwood, ON L0C 1A0

Alberta Nurseries & Seeds
    PO Box 20
    Bowden, AL T0M 0K0

Prairie Garden Seeds
    PO Box 118
    Cochin, SK S0M 0L0

Terra Edibles
    Box 164
    Foxboro, ON K0K 2B0

Mapple Farm
    RR #1
    Hillsborough, NB E0A 1X0

Salt Spring Seeds
  PO Box 444, Ganges
  Salt Spring Island, BC V8K 2W1

MEAT AND POULTRY

WHILE FOOD derived from genetically engineered animals is not currently being sold in supermarkets—except for dairy products coming from diary cows injected with the genetically engineered milk hormone rBGH—experimental transgenic pigs, cattle, and fish are expected to be commercialized soon. But the real concern right now is with animal feed. Up to 80 percent of genetically engineered grain is being utilized for animal feed.[7]

In response to public concerns about the safety of meat, eggs and poultry in general, a burgeoning market is evolving in GE-free, organic/free-range/no hormone meat. In January 1999, for the first time, the U.S. Department of Agriculture allowed meat to be labeled as organic. The rule allows organic certification agencies to certify as "organic" meat produced by farmers that do not use pesticide-treated feed, growth hormones, or antibiotics. Additionally, current organic rules require that meat and poultry are raised on organic feed, without the use of antibiotics or growth hormones, that the animals have access to fresh water and pasture, and that there is a manure management plan.

However, just because meat is labeled organic at the present time doesn't mean that the livestock it comes from hasn't been fed GE corn or soybeans or other GE-derived feed ingredients. This statement by Laura's Lean Beef on genetically engineered feed, outlines some of the problems involved:

> Laura's Lean Beef is opposed to the use of GMOs in our livestock feeds. We ask our farmers not to plant genetically engineered corn and soybeans. However, at times some of our farmers must purchase corn and soybeans from commercial silos. As part of our program we check

this feed for pesticide residues, in addition to antibiotics and growth hormones. Since there is no labeling for GMOs, and at present no system for keeping genetically engineered grain separate from traditional grain, we cannot ensure that all our cattle feed is free of GMOs.[8]

While there is only a limited supply of organic meat currently on the market, it is a rapidly growing segment of the organic market. And the growing opposition to GE in the U.S. will undoubtedly fuel an even greater demand for organic meat labeled as GE-free. New proposed federal regulations on organic standards released by the USDA in March, 2000 will require all certified organic animals to be fed 100 percent organic feed—thereby excluding all GE-derived feed.

A recent survey done by Greenpeace in the United Kingdom found that major food retailers are rushing to source meat, eggs, and dairy products from non-GM fed animals to counter widespread customer concern. Tesco, the largest food retailer in the U.K., has already written to major international animal feed suppliers, Cargill and Archer Daniel Midlands, informing them of their intention to eliminate genetically engineered ingredients in animal feed.[9]

Besides your local co-op or supermarket there are numerous other companies selling organic meat that you can contact directly. See chapter 10 for a list of companies selling organic meat and poultry.

WHO OFFERS RBGH-FREE MILK?

SINCE THE recombinant Bovine Growth Hormone (rBGH) was introduced onto the market in 1993, a limited percentage of the U.S. milk supply has come from cows injected with the hormone. Since the milk of many different cows is routinely co-mingled in bulk tanks at most of the nation's dairies, this means that the majority of non-organic dairy products probably contain at least trace levels of rBGH. While Monsanto, the maker of rBGH, claims that up to one-third of U.S. cows have been injected,[10] critics of the drug believe the actual figure is more like 5–7 percent. In response to rBGH's introduction into the milk business, several hundred companies now require written affidavits from their milk suppliers that no rBGH was injected into the cows, and label the milk as rBGH-free. Approximately 10 percent of fluid milk in the U.S. is now labeled rBGH-free.

Others have capitalized on the growing market niche of organic milk—which is guaranteed to be GE-free since organic certification prohibits the use of rBGH. Since the introduction of rBGH, sales of organic milk has skyrocketed. For instance, sales grew from $16 million in 1996, to $31 million in 1997.[11]

Ben & Jerry's Homemade Inc. takes steps to ensure that the milk in its ice cream does not come from cows injected with recombinant Bovine Growth Hormone. The company is also making sure that brownies and other ingredients are not made from genetically engineered ingredients.

All dairy products made from sheep or goat's milk are rBGH-free because the drug is not used with these animals. Recombinant Bovine Growth Hormone is not approved for use in Canada, the European Union, New Zealand, and Australia. Cheeses and other dairy products from any of these countries are rBGH-free.

Below is a partial list, put together by Rural Vermont and Mothers & Others for a Livable Planet, of milk and dairy companies that have pledged that their milk does not come from cows injected with the Bovine Growth Hormone. The first section lists companies with organic dairy products; the second section lists companies with rBGH-free (but not necessarily organic) products. Those marked with "*" are small family farms.

THESE MILK and dairy companies carry some or all organic products.

- Alta Dena Organics (cheese), City of Industry, CA, 800-535-1369, available nationwide.
- Bart's Homemade Low-Fat Organic Ice Cream, Greenfield, MA, 413-774-7438, available in Massachusetts, New Hampshire, Connecticut, and at their own store in Greenfield.
- Brookside Farm* (milk and cream), Westminster, MA, 978-874-2695, available in Massachusetts.
- Butternut Farms* (cheese), NY, 607-783-2392,www.butternutfarms.com, available in the Northeast and by mail order.
- Butterworks Farm* (yogurt, cream, cheese, cottage cheese), Westfield, VT, 802-744-6855, available in the Northeast and at the farm; cheese also available by mail order.
- Cascadian Farm (frozen yogurt, ice cream), Sedro-Wooley, WA, 800-624-4123, available nationwide.
- Cedar Grove Organic Cheese, Plain, WI, 608-546-5284, www.familyfarm.org, available in the Upper Midwest, at their own store in Plain, and by mail order (800-275-8354).
- Echo Spring Dairy (organic line) (milk, sour cream, cottage cheese), Eugene, OR, 541-753-7331, available in Idaho, Oregon, and northern California.
- Greenbank Farms Cheese (organic line), Stonefelt Cheese Co., Preston, WA, 425/222-5500, available on the West Coast, in the Northwest, and at their own store in Preston.
- Hart-to-Hart Farm* (cheese and licensed raw milk), Albion, ME, 207-437-2441, available at the farm and at farmers' markets throughout central Maine (call for locations).
- Hawthorne Valley Farm* (cheese, yogurt, and quark cheese), Ghent, NY, 518-672-7500, available on the East Coast. Raw

milk and cheese also available at their own local store and at the Union Square Farmers' Market in New York City.

- Horizon Organic Dairy (milk, chocolate milk, cream, whipped cream, yogurt, cheese, butter, sour cream, cottage cheese, cream cheese), Boulder, CO, 888-494-3020, available nationwide.
- Kimberton Hills Farm* (licensed raw milk), Kimberton, PA, available at Kimberton Whole Foods Store (610-935-1444) and at the farm (610-935-0314).
- Lifeline Farms Cheese*, Victor, MT, available on the West Coast. For store locations, call Mountain Peoples, 800-679-8735, cfs.Colorado.edu/co-op/mountain.html.
- Morningland Dairy Cheese*, Mountain View, MO, 417-469-3817, available nationwide and by mail order.
- Natural by Nature (cheese, cream, buttermilk, eggnog, ice cream, butter, yogurt, cream cheese, milk, pudding), Sunnydale Farms, Brooklyn, NY, 718-257-7600, available on the East Coast and in the Midwest.
- Nezinscot Farm* (cow's or goat's milk, cheese, butter), Turner, ME, 207-225-3231, available at their own store in Turner; cheese available by mail order.
- Organic Cow of Vermont (milk, chocolate milk, sour cream, cottage cheese, butter, cream, eggnog), Chelsea, VT, 800-769-9693, available on the East Coast.
- Organic Valley* (milk, cheese, butter, cream cheese, cottage cheese, sour cream, cream, powdered milk), La Farge, WI, 608-625-2600, www.organicvalley.com, available nationwide.
- Ranovael Organic Dairy* (cheese, butter), DePere, WI, cheese available by mail order through Greener Pastures, 920-338-8717. Both products are available at their own store in DePere, 920-336-2820.
- Seven Stars Farm* (yogurt), Phoenixville, PA 610-935-1949, available in the East and Midwest.
- Stonyfield Farms (organic line) (yogurt and ice cream), Londonderry, NH, 603-437-4040, available nationwide.

- Straus Family Creamery* (milk, butter, yogurt, cheese), Marshall, CA, 415-663-5464, www.strausmilk.com, available in California, Arizona, and New Mexico.
- Wisconsin Organics* (milk, cheese, butter), Bonduel, WI, 715-758-2280, available nationwide and at their own retail store in Bonduel.

RBGH-FREE (BUT NOT ORGANIC) BRANDS

THESE MILK and dairy companies carry some or all rBGH-free products.

- Alta Dena (milk, buttermilk, chocolate milk, eggnog, cream, sour cream, yogurt, natural select butter, ice cream, cottage cheese, and all cheeses except for cream cheese), City of Industry, CA, 800-MILK123, available nationwide.
- Balance Rock Farm (milk), Berlin, MA, 978-838-2024, available at their farm store in Berlin.
- Ben & Jerry's Ice Cream, S. Burlington, VT, 802-846-1500, www.benjerry.com/ca/, available nationwide.
- Biazzo Dairy Products (cheese), Riverfield, NJ, 201-941-6800, available nationwide.
- Blythedale Farm Cheese*, Corinth, VT, 802-439-6575, available in the Northeast.
- Booth Brothers Dairy (milk, cream, chocolate milk, eggnog), Barre, VT, 802-476-6605, available in Vermont and New Hampshire.
- Brigham's Ice Cream, Arlington, MA, 800-Brighams, www.brighams.com, available in the Northeast.
- Brown Cow Farm (milk and yogurt), Antioch, CA, 925-757-9209, www.wholemilkyogurt.com, available nationwide.
- Calabro Cheese Corp., East Haven, CT, 203-469-1311, www.calabrocheese.com, available on the East and West Coasts and in Ohio.

- Cedar Grove's Family Farmer Cheeses*, Plain, WI, 608-546-5284, www.familyfarm.org, available in the Upper Midwest, at their own store in Plain, and by mail order (800-200-6020).
- Clover Stornetta Farms (milk, cheese, sour cream, yogurt), Petaluma, CA, 800-237-3315, www.clo-the-cow.com, available in northern California.
- Crescent Creamery (milk), Pittsfield, MA, 800-221-6455, available in the Northeast.
- Crooked Creek Farm Dairy (milk, ice cream), Romeo, MI, 810-752-6095, available at farm dairy store and at select stores in southeast Michigan.
- Crowley Cheese of Vermont, Healdville, VT, 802-259-2210, www.newenglandcheese.com/website/crowley/index2.htm, available nationwide and by mail order.
- Derle Farms (milk with "no rBST" label only), Brooklyn, NY, 718/257-2040, available in New York and New Jersey.
- Dorchester Ice Cream, Boston, MA, 617-282-9600, available in the Northeast.
- Egg Farm Dairy (butter, cheese, ice cream, cream), Peekskill, NY, 800-CREAMERY, available at their local retail store, by mail order, and nationwide at gourmet food stores.
- Erivan Dairy Yogurt*, Oreland, PA, 215-887-2009, available on the East Coast and in the Midwest.
- Farmland Dairies (milk, chocolate milk, cream), Wallington, NJ, 800-327-9522, available on the east coast.
- Franklin County Cream (Bagel Factory, Shaw's Cream Cheese, Bruegger's Bagels Cream Cheese—Eastern US only, All Seasons Kitchen, Lombardi's—Cream Cheese and Mascarpone, Vermont Butter and Cheese—Mascarpone, Enosburg Falls, VT, 802-933-4338, www.franklinfoods.com, available nationwide.
- Golden Guernsey Dairy (milk), and Morning Glory Dairy (milk), from Foremost Farms, Baraboo, WI, 608-356-8316, available in Wisconsin and northern Illinois.

- Grafton Village Cheese, Grafton, VT, 800-472-3866, 802-843-2221, www.graftonvillagecheese.com, available nationwide and by mail order.
- Great Hill Dairy (cheese), Marion, MA, 508-748-2208, www.greathillblue.com, available by mail order or nationwide at gourmet stores.
- Hatchland Dairy* (milk, chocolate milk, eggnog, cream), N. Haverhill, NH, 603/787-2388, available in New Hampshire and Vermont.
- Jilbert's Dairy (milk, ice cream), Marquette, MI, 906-225-1363, available in Michigan upper peninsula through Wisconsin border.
- Joseph Farms Cheese, Joseph Gallo, Atwater, CA, 209-394-7984, www.josephfarms.com, available in the Northwest, Southwest, South, and Hawaii.
- Kate's Homemade Butter, Old Orchard Beach, ME, 207-934-5134, available nationwide.
- Kemp's Select (milk), Kemp's Marigold Foods, Minneapolis, MN, 800/726-6455, available in Minnesota, Wisconsin, and Iowa.
- Lifetime Dairy Cheese, Lifeline Food Co., Seaside, CA, 831-899-5040, www.lifetimefatfree.com, available nationwide.
- McNamara Dairy* (milk, chocolate milk, eggnog, cream, whipped cream), West Lebanon, NH, 603-298-6666, available in New Hampshire and Vermont.
- Monument Farms* (milk, cottage cheese, buttermilk, cream), Middlebury, VT, 802-545-2119, available in Vermont and at their own store in Weybridge, VT.
- North Farm Cooperative* (cheese), Madison, WI, 800-236-5880, 608-241-2667, www.northfarm-coop.com, available nationwide and by mail order.
- Oberweiss Dairy (milk and ice cream), Aurora, IL, 630-897-6600, available in Illinois.

- Orb Weaver Farm* (cheese), New Haven, VT, 802-877-3755, available in Vermont, by mail order, at the farm, and at Murray's Cheese Shop in New York City.
- Pollard Dairy (milk, chocolate milk, whipped cream), Norway, MI, 906-563-8815, Michigan upper peninsula, northeastern Wisconsin.
- Rustling Winds Creamery (cheese, milk but bring your own container), Falls Village, CT, 860-824-7084, available at their farm store; cheese available by mail order.
- Salemville Cheese, North Farm Cooperative, Madison, WI, 800-236-5880, nationwide and by mail order.
- Shelburne Farms Farmhouse Cheddar Cheese*, Shelburne, VT, 802-985-8686, available nationwide, by mail order, and at their own farm-site store.
- Stonyfield Farms (yogurt, frozen yogurt, ice cream), Londonderry, NH, 603-437-5050, www.stonyfield.com, available nationwide.
- Sugarbush Farm* (cheese), Woodstock, VT, 800-281-1757, available in the Northeast and by mail order.
- Thomas Dairy (milk, cream, eggnog, chocolate milk, butter, sour cream, yogurt, buttermilk), Rutland, VT, 802-773-6788, available in central Vermont.
- Vermont Family Farms* (milk), Vermont Milk Producers, Whiting, VT, 802-897-2769, available in Vermont, New Hampshire, Massachusetts, and upstate New York.
- Westby Cooperative Creamery* (cottage cheese, sour cream, french onion dip, butter, cheese), Westby, WI, 800-492-9282, www.westbycreamery.com, available in Wisconsin, Minnesota, Iowa, and Illinois and at their own store in Westby; cheese available by mail order.
- Wilcox Dairy (milk, ice cream), Manchester, VT, 800-262-1223, available in Vermont, New Hampshire, Massachusetts, and in upstate New York.

IAMS CO., the Ohio-based pet food manufacturer, recently told its grain suppliers it would no longer accept genetically engineered corn for use in its premium dog and cat chows unless the corn varieties were among the few approved by the European Union. Unfortunately, the same cannot be said for Alpo—which has tested positive for genetically engineered ingredients in its dog food, and Purina which has said, "Because genetically modified grain and grain products constitute a significant portion of the supply of grain available throughout the U.S. for both human and pet foods, it is likely that our pet food products contain genetically modified grain."[12]

8

FOODS AND BRANDS YOU SHOULD BUY AND WHERE YOU CAN FIND THEM

AS AN American consumer, you have been placed in a very difficult situation if you want to avoid genetically engineered food. If there is no labeling, and conventional foods are mixed together with genetically engineered foods, how do you know what to avoid? Is it all simply luck of the draw? The situation leaves even the most careful consumer feeling vulnerable. Without question, it can be difficult to completely eliminate genetically engineered foods and ingredients from your diet. But, you can take several important steps that will dramatically reduce your exposure to genetically engineered food. By doing so, you will be supporting the type of farming that is decidedly against genetic engineering.

In order to buy GE-free foods, you'll have to play very close attention to where your food comes from, how it is produced, and who is producing it. You need to arm yourself with the best information available in order to make smart choices in the marketplace.

FIRST LINE OF DEFENSE—GO ORGANIC!

TEN YEARS ago, it was hard to find organic food in the marketplace. Organic food was considered an inconsequential segment of the food industry, to be found mostly in small co-ops, with little selection and expensive prices. But all that has changed. A 1999 Food Marketing Institute study found that organic and natural foods are available at approximately 73 percent of grocery stores and supermarkets. And the increase in accessibility is being driven by consumer demand. The FMI study also found that more than 50 percent of consumers seek out products labeled "organic", and 63 percent look for products labeled "natural."[1]

The organic food industry is the fastest growing sector of the food industry. Since 1989, it has grown 20–25 percent a year and is now estimated at over $5 billion a year in sales. This is still a small percentage of the $346.1 billion in supermarket sales in 1999. But Packaged Facts, a New York City-based market research firm, is predicting that sales of organic foods and beverages will increase by more than 150 percent to $6.6 billion by the end of 2000.[2]

About 6,600 U.S. farmers are now certified organic (with an estimated 1.3 million acres of certified organic cropland), with an additional 15,000 running trials on organic plots, according to the Organic Farming Research Foundation. The number of organic farmers is increasing by 12 percent a year, according to the USDA. These farms help to make organic food available at 400 co-ops, hundreds of farmers' markets, buying clubs, and even mainstream supermarkets. In fact, more than 30 percent of organics are now sold through mass-market grocers, according to the Organic Trade Association's 1998 Manufacturers' Market Survey.[3]

The growth in organic industry has been driven almost entirely by consumers and organic farmers—with almost no help from the government. Funding figures from the USDA's Agricultural Research Service show that only about $1 million of the current $800 million research budget is spent on organic projects, compared with $30.7 million on genetic engineering.[4]

There is good reason to believe that a major contributor to the organic industry's recent growth is the introduction of GE foods. "Organics have benefited, in the short run anyway, from GMOs because the only way to verify that you're not eating genetically modified organisms is to buy organic foods," says Karen Klonsky, an economist in the Department of Agricultural and Resource Economics at the University of California, Davis.[5]

The attraction to organic food is simple. Organic food is grown in a natural, environmentally-safe manner without the use of synthetic pesticides, herbicides, or fertilizers. Instead, farmers rely on traditional farming methods that have been utilized for centuries—including crop rotation, the use of beneficial insects, composted manure as fertilizer—and a lot of hard work. Organic farming follows a philosophy of working with nature instead of working against it.

An added benefit of eating organic food is that it just might be more nutritious than conventional food. Although research on this issue is only just beginning in earnest, University of Copenhagen researchers have found that organic food contains more secondary metabolites than conventionally grown plants. Secondary metabolite are substances which form part of the plants' immune systems, and which also help to fight cancer in humans. Those same studies indicate that organic crops have a measurably higher levels of vitamins.[6]

This new evidence on the nutritional value of organic food appears in stark contrast to the apparent nutrient declines on conventional food. In an analysis of USDA nutrient data from 1975 to 1997, the Kushi Institute of Becket, MA found that the average calcium levels in twelve fresh vegetables declined 27 percent; iron levels dropped 37 percent; vitamin A levels 21 percent, and vitamin C levels 30 percent. A similar analysis of British nutrient data from 1930 to 1980 published in the *British Food Journal* found that in 20 vegetables, the average calcium content had declined 19 percent; iron 22 percent; and potassium 14 percent.[7]

And most importantly for the purposes of this book, organic food production as enforced by all forty-four different certification bodies in the U.S., forbids the use of genetically engineered foods. Newly developed rules for organic food by the USDA will also explicitly forbid the use of genetically engineered ingredients. However, it should be pointed out that there are still small possibilities that organic food could become contaminated with genetically engineered material. Processed or packaged organic foods can include up to 5 percent of non-organic ingredients. Those ingredients could be genetically engineered if the company has not ensured that its sources are not using genetically engineered crops. More and more organic companies are now taking steps to ensure that 100 percent of their ingredient sources are not genetically engineered.

In addition, organic fields are under constant threat from genetic contamination or drift from neighboring farms. Remember the Terra Prima case detailed in chapter 2? In addition, a major organic farm in Britain was forced to decertify as organic, after genetically engineered material drifted onto the farm. To combat this potential problem, more and more organic and natural food companies are having their sources and food tested to check for cases of drift.

TOP 10 REASONS TO BUY ORGANIC

1. **Protect future generations.** The average child receives four times more exposure than an adult to at least eight widely used cancer-causing pesticides in food. The food choices you make now will impact your child's' health in the future.

2. **Prevent soil erosion.** The Soil Conservation Service estimates that more than 3 billion tons of topsoil are eroded from United States croplands each year.

That means soil is eroding seven times faster than it is being built up naturally. Soil is the foundation of the food chain in organic farming. But in conventional farming the soil is used more as a medium for holding plants in a vertical position so they can be chemically fertilized. As a result, American farms are suffering from the worst soil erosion in history.

3. **Protect water quality.** Water makes up two-thirds of our body mass and covers three-fourths of the planet. Despite its importance, the Environmental Protection Agency (EPA) estimates pesticides—some cancer-causing—contaminate the groundwater in 38 states, polluting the primary source of drinking water for more than half the country's population.

4. **Save energy.** American farms have changed drastically in the last three generations, from family-based small businesses dependent on human energy to large-scale factory farms highly dependent on fossil fuels.

   Modern farming uses more petroleum than any other single industry, consuming 12 percent of the country's total energy supply. More energy is now used to produce synthetic fertilizers than to till, cultivate, and harvest all the crops in the United States.

   Organic farming is still mainly based on labor-intensive practices such as weeding by hand and using green manures and crop covers rather than synthetic fertilizers to build up soil. Organic produce also tends to travel fewer miles from field to table.

5. **Keep chemicals off your plate.** Many pesticides approved for use by the EPA were registered long before extensive research linking these chemicals to cancer and other diseases had been established. Now the EPA considers that 60 percent of all herbicides, 90 percent of all fungicides and 30 percent of all insecticides are carcinogenic. A 1987 National Academy of Sciences report estimated that pesticides might cause an extra 1.4 million cancer cases among Americans over their lifetimes. The bottom line is that pesticides are poisons designed to kill living organisms, and can also be harmful to humans. In addition to cancer, pesticides are implicated in birth defects, nerve damage and genetic mutation.

6. **Protect farm worker health.** A National Cancer Institute study found that farmers exposed to herbicides had a six times greater risk than non-farmers of contracting cancer.

   In California, reported pesticide poisonings among farm workers have risen an average of 14 percent a year since 1973, and doubled between 1975 and 1985. Field workers suffer the highest rates of occupational illness in the state. Farm worker health also is a serious problem in developing nations, where pesticide use can be poorly regulated. An estimated 1 million people are poisoned annually by pesticides.

7. **Help small farmers.** Although more and more large-scale farms are making the conversion to organic practices, most organic farms are small independently owned and operated family farms of less than 100 acres.

   It's estimated that the United States has lost more than 650,000 family farms in the past decade. And with the U.S. Department of Agriculture predicting that half of this country's farm production will come from 1 percent of farms by the year 2000, organic farming could be one of the few survival tactics left for family farms.

8. **Support a true economy.** Although organic foods might seem more expensive than conventional foods, conventional food prices do not reflect hidden costs borne by taxpayers, including billions of dollars annually in federal subsidies. Other hidden costs include pesticide regulation and testing, hazardous waste disposal and clean-up, and environmental damage.

   As health writer Gary Null has pointed out, if you add in the real environmental and social costs of irrigation to a head of lettuce, its price can range between $2 and $3.

9. **Promote biodiversity.** Mono-cropping is the practice of planting large plots of land with the same crop year after year. While this approach tripled farm production between 1950 and 1970, the lack of natural diversity of plant life has left the soil lacking in natural minerals and nutrients. To replace the nutrients, chemical fertilizers are used often in increasing amounts.

   Single crops are also much more susceptible to pests, making farmers more reliant on pesticides. Despite a tenfold increase in the use of pesticides between 1947 and 1974, crop losses due to insects have doubled—partly because some insects have become genetically resistant to certain pesticides.

10. **Taste better flavor.** There's a good reason why many chefs use organic foods in their recipes—they taste better! Organic farming starts with the nourishment of the soil, which eventually leads to the nourishment of the plant and, ultimately, our palates.

    Source: Committee for Sustainable Agriculture

HOW DO YOU KNOW IT'S ORGANIC?

FINDING OUT whether a food is organic will become a lot simpler once the new USDA national rules for organic are fully implemented—projected to be January 2002. Organic food producers are currently required to be certified by official, independent agencies to make sure they are following procedures consistent with organic food production. However, there are over 40 different organic certification agencies nation-wide. Eleven of the certification programs are state-run, while the rest are private or nongovernmental certification agencies. The precise specifications for qualifying as "organic" vary slightly among the different certification agencies. However, most analysts agree that all of the U.S. certification bodies currently operate at a high standard that consumers can trust. The new national organic food rules established by the USDA will unify all certification agencies to work under one standard. And the organic label will be uniform as well.

Under the proposed new USDA organic rules, products labeled as "organic" must be composed of 95 percent organically produced ingredients. Processed products with 50 percent to 95 percent organic ingredients must use the phrase "made with organic ingredients." If a product is less than half organic, the organic items may be listed only in the ingredient list on the side panel.

Food is certified organic only when the certification agency is satisfied that the farm is meeting its standards for organic food production—ie, not using toxic pesticides, genetically-engineered crops or inputs, hormones, antibiotics etc. If the food is not labeled "certified organic," then it has not been officially approved by these organic certification bodies. However, thousands of small farmers in the U.S. do produce genuine organic products, even if they can't afford to pay certification fees.

Until the USDA organic rule goes into effect, it is good to become familiar with the current U.S. organic certification agencies. If you regularly buy organic food, you might recognize them:

PRIVATE ORGANIC CERTIFICATION ORGANIZATIONS:

- Appalachian Mushroom Growers Association
- California Certified Organic Farmers (CCOF)
- Carolina Farm Stewardship Association (CFSA)
- The Demeter Association, Inc.
- Farm Verified Organic, Inc. (FVO)
- Florida Organic Growers & Consumers, Inc. (FOGC)
- Georgia Organic Growers Association (GOGA)
- Global Organic Alliance
- Hawaii Bio-organic Growers Association (HBGA)
- Hawaii Organic Farmers Association (HOFA)
- Indiana Certified Organic
- Kauai Organic Growers Association (KOGA)
- Living Farms, Inc.
- Maine Organic Farmers & Gardeners Association (MOFGA)
- Mountain State Organic Growers & Buyers Association (MSOGBA)
- Northeast Organic Farming Association—Connecticut (NOFA-CT)
- Northeast Organic Farming Association—Massachusetts (NOFA-MA)
- Northeast Organic Farming Association—New Jersey (NOFA-NJ)
- Northeast Organic Farming Association—New York (NOFA-NY)
- Northeast Organic Farming Association—Vermont (NOFA-VT)
- Ohio Ecological Food & Farming Association (OEFFA)
- Oregon Tilth Certified Organically Grown (OTCOG)
- Organic Certification Services, Inc. (OCS)
- Organic Crop Improvement Association (OCIA)
- Organic Forum International
- Organic Growers & Buyers Association (OGBA)

- Organic Growers of Michigan
- Organic Verification Organization of North America (OVONA)
- Pennsylvania Certified Organic
- Quality Assurance International (QAI)
- Scientific Certification Systems (SCS)
- Tennessee Land Stewardship Association (TLSA)
- Tidewater Organic Growers Association (TOGA)
- United States Assurance Laboratories (USAL)
- Vermont Maple Sugarmaker's Association, Inc. (VMSA)
- Virginia Biological Farmers Association (VABF)

STATES THAT HAVE CERTIFICATION PROGRAMS—USUALLY THROUGH THE STATE AGRICULTURE DEPARTMENT

- Colorado
- Idaho
- Indiana
- Iowa
- Kentucky
- Louisiana
- Maryland
- New Hampshire
- New Mexico
- Texas
- Washington

Take notice that foods labeled as "natural" are not certified as organic by any of these agencies. "Natural" simply means that a food or beverage has been produced without any artificial additives or preservatives. This is definitely a plus for consumers because this makes it easier to read the ingredients of natural products. However, just because a product is labeled "natural" does not mean it is GE-free. A growing number of natural food companies are taking steps to ensure that their ingredients sources are not genetically engineered. So, look to see if the natural product has also labeled itself GE-free.

WHERE CAN YOU FIND ORGANIC FOOD? START AT THE SUPERMARKET

ORGANIC FOOD is no longer relegated strictly to the realm of neighborhood food co-ops, buying clubs and farmers' markets. It can now be found in most major supermarkets, although you may have to look hard to find it—and the selection may not be adequate. Major supermarkets like Safeway, Krogers, Albertson's, Winn-Dixie and Cub Foods now have organic sections, and are becoming more and more responsive to consumer demands for greater variety and quality. If the organic/natural food aisle isn't big enough, talk with the store manager, and make sure to keep buying organic. These supermarket chains track every purchase and are finely attuned to consumer trends.

In fact, the Minnesota-based Organic Alliance is working closely with a number of these mainstream supermarkets to make organic food products more available at some of the nation's largest supermarket chain—Kroger's, A&P, Wegmans, Publix, Byerly's, Lunds, Pratt Foods, King Soopers, and Food Emporium. An April 2000 promotion by the Organic Alliance targeted 500 supermarkets in cities in New York, New Jersey, Connecticut, Colorado, Minnesota, Wisconsin, Florida, Georgia, Illinois, Oklahoma, Oregon, California, and North and South Carolina.

But beyond the giant conventional supermarket chains, there are a growing number of specialty "organic and natural" food stores. The industry leaders are Whole Foods and Wild Oats. As we discussed in chapter 7, both Whole Foods and Wild Oats have pledged to make their own brand-name products genetically-engineered free. The Austin, Texas-based Whole Foods Market Inc.

operates 103 stores (some under the name Fresh Fields) in 22 states. Wild Oats, based in Boulder, and operates 110-stores. They are the first major supermarket chains in America to ban genetically engineered ingredients in their brand name products.

JOIN A FOOD CO-OP

THE NUMBER and size of consumer food co-ops continues to grow in the U.S. There are now an estimated 350 co-ops located around the country, with over $500 million in annual sales—some co-ops now rival mainstream supermarket chains in terms of size and sales volume.[8] Food co-ops generally offer a full range of organic and natural food, and are set up to directly serve the needs and preferences of their members and customers. Co-ops are run democratically, and when you join, you become part-owner. Food co-ops are non-profits, and often run at least partly on the power of volunteers. As a member of a co-op, you are usually entitled to certain discounts and sometimes even rebates at the end of the year. In the old days of co-ops, people qualified as members by volunteering time at the co-op. This concept is still alive at many U.S. co-ops, but most also offer the option of simply paying for membership. Generally, it is not necessary for you to become a formal member of a food co-op in order to shop at the store.

The best resource list for food co-ops is the National Co-op Directory, put out by the Co-op Network.

Co-op Network
Box 57
Randolph, VT 05060
802-234-9293

Another listing of co-ops on the Internet is the U.S. and Canadian Directory of Co-ops, which allows you to search by state to find a co-op near you: www.purefood.org/coopindex.htm

OWN A SHARE OF THE FARM—COMMUNITY SUPPORTED AGRICULTURE

A GREAT way to get fresh organic produce and other food items—and support organic and small farms in your area—is by joining a Community Supported Agriculture (CSA) program. The concept of CSA programs, having begun only in the mid-1980s, is relatively new to U.S. agriculture. CSAs originated in the 1960s in Japan, where a group of women concerned about the increase in food imports and the diminishing number of farms began to buy directly from local farms. The arrangement, called "teikei" in Japanese, translates to "putting the farmers' face on food."

When you buy food at the supermarket, it is estimated that your food has travelled an average of 1,500 miles from the farm to the market shelf. Almost every state in the U.S. buys 85–90 percent of its food from some place else, according to a University of Massachusetts analysis. Enrolling in a CSA can help put you in better touch with where your food comes from and let you discover foods being grown seasonally in your state or community. CSA's can dramatically reduce the "food miles" of the items in your pantry and promote local and regional food production.

There are currently more than 1,000 CSA farms in the U.S. and Canada with most located near urban centers in New England, the Mid-Atlantic states, and the Great Lakes region.[9] A growing number are being established in other areas around the country, including on the West Coast.

A CSA works similar to buying stock in a company. To join a CSA, you buy a share of the harvest. As a shareholder, you receive a portion of the food produced each year from the farm. The amount you receive depends on the extent of the farm's bounty. In addition to owning part of the farm's produce, you also have the opportunity to visit the farm and work on it to better understand exactly how the food is grown. At some CSAs, you can even work off a portion of your share. Spending a day learning about where your food comes from, the hard work needed to grow the food, and the remarkable skill and knowledge of your local farmer can be a great learning experience for adults and children alike.

In most cases, CSAs extend over the entire growing season in your region. Members sign up and buy their share at the beginning of the growing season—usually in one lump sum, although sometimes installments are available. Most CSAs offer a diversity of vegetables, fruits, and herbs in season; some provide a full array of farm produce, including shares in eggs, meat, milk, baked goods, and even firewood. And every week you will pick up, or have delivered to a distribution point, a box full of fresh food produced at the farm the previous week. As crops rotate throughout the season, weekly shares vary by size and types of produce, reflecting local growing seasons and conditions. Most shares are designed to meet the produce needs of a family of four for one week. But in many cases, what you get is far too much food for one family or household, and you'll find yourself either learning to can or preserve your surplus, or else sharing your weekly CSA bounty with friends or co-workers.

To tap into an increasing demand from consumers for fresh food alternatives, USDA's Sustainable Agriculture Network (SAN) has assembled a list of CSA farms nationwide. Available in print as well as on the World Wide Web, the list of more than 450 farms offers names and contact information for CSA operations in almost every state. To access the new CSA list, see www.sare.org/san/csa/index.htm, where you can search by state. Farmers and consumers can receive lists of CSA farms in their states by writing to CSA/CSREES, 1400 Independence Ave., S.W., Stop 2207, Washington, DC 20250–2207.

WHY IS COMMUNITY SUPPORTED AGRICULTURE IMPORTANT?

■ CSA's direct marketing gives farmers and growers the fairest return on their products.

- CSA keeps food dollars in the local community and contributes to the maintenance and establishment of regional food production.
- CSA encourages communication and cooperation among farmers.
- With a "guaranteed market" for their produce, farmers can invest their time in doing the best job they can rather than looking for buyers.
- CSA supports the biodiversity of a given area and the diversity of agriculture through the preservation of small farms producing a wide variety of crops.
- CSA creates opportunity for dialogue between farmers and consumers.
- CSA creates a sense of social responsibility and stewardship of local land.
- CSA puts "the farmers face on food" and increases understanding of how, where, and by whom our food is grown.

Source: UMass Extension Agroecology Program.

MEET YOUR FARMER AT THE MARKET

ANOTHER GREAT way to find non-GE organic food is at farmers' markets. The U.S. has seen an explosion of farmers' markets in the last ten years. USDA's National Farmers Market Directory listed just 656 in 1994. Now, the USDA estimates there are close to 3,000 farmers' markets—involving over 10,000 farmers—around the country.

While the approximately $1 billion in farmers' market sales is a fraction of the $300 billion in U.S. agricultural sales, the small figure represents direct sales from farmers to consumers—with no corporate middle man.[10]

These markets can usually be found in urban areas—where farmers outside the city have come to a common location to sell their produce. For example, in New York City, Greenmarket now runs 28 different farmers' markets throughout the city.

Farmers' markets give you an opportunity to actually meet the farmer growing your food. While you're there, you can ask him or her about their growing practices. Many farmers at farmers' markets are using organic methods and most are not using genetically engineered seeds—but you should always ask if the farmer is certified organic.

Farmers' markets are also a big part of the Women, Infants, and Children (WIC) Program. In 1992, WIC established its Farmers Market Program to provide fresh, nutritious, unprepared foods, such as fruit and vegetables, from farmers to people who are nutritionally at risk and to expand the awareness and use of farmers markets by consumers. The use of food stamps at farmers' markets nationwide is huge—estimates range from $75 million to $100 million annually, according to the USDA.

Additionally, sales from farmers' markets to school meals programs are being promoted by USDA's Agricultural Marketing Service, Rural Development, and Food and Nutrition Service in California, Florida, Georgia, and North Carolina.

USDA makes it easy to find a listing of the farmers' markets in your state. Go to Internet site www.ams.usda.gov/farmersmarkets and click on a picture of your state to bring up an alphabetical listing.

JOIN A BUYING CLUB

WHOLESALE BUYING clubs are yet another resource for organic and natural products dry goods. Thousands of organic and natural food buying clubs have now sprung up across the country—both in rural and urban areas. The eight wholesale distributors listed below deliver food to buying clubs as well as supplying retail consumer co-ops and also supply co-ops. Buying clubs are groups of people who join together and purchase foods and other grocery items in bulk at considerable savings. By buying in bulk or combining their order, buying clubs can often save you 10–50 percent off retail prices on organic and natural food products. This basically means that you can buy the highest quality organic food through your buying club at prices cheaper than conventional foods in your local supermarket. A buying club can be as small as one or two house-holds within a city block or as large as 1,000 households in a hun-dred mile radius. Many times, buying clubs are informal organiza-tions made up of friends, family, co-workers, church groups, and other associations. You may also be able to join an existing buying club in your area. Contact one of the wholesalers below to find out whether there is a buying club in your area.

Blooming Prairie Warehouse
   2340 Heinz Road
   Iowa City, IA 52240
   Fax: 319-337-4592
   Phone: 319-337-6448
   Web site: www.bpco-op/index.html

Blooming Prairie Natural Foods,
   510 Kasota Ave SE
   Minneapolis,MN
   Phone: 612-378-9774
   Web site: www.bpco-op.com/index.html

North Farm Cooperative
   204 Regas Road
   Madison, WI 53714
   Fax: 608-241-0688
   Phone:1-800-236-5880
   Web site: www.northfarm-coop.com
   Serves Indiana, OH, MN, WI, KY, MO, IL, MI, ND, WY

Northeast Cooperatives
   90 Technology Drive
   PO Box 8188
   Brattleboro, VT 05304-8188
   Phone: 802-257-5856
   Web site: www.northeastcoop.com

■ ■ ■

215 Williams St
Chelsea, MA 02150
Phone: 800-736-9032 (only for NE area)
Web site: (see above)
Serves New England, PA, NY, and NJ

Federation of Ohio River Cooperatives
320 E Outerbelt St
Columbus, OH 43213
Fax: 614-861-7638
Phone: 614-861-2446, 1-888-936-9648
Web site: www.forcwarehouse.com
Serves MI, IN OH, PA, WV, VA, NC, SC, GA, TN, and KY

Frontier Natural Products Coop
2990 Wilderness Pl Suite 200
Boulder, CO 80301
Fax: 303-449-8139
Phone: 303-449-8137
Web site: www.frontiercoop.com

Ozark Cooperative Warehouse
Box 1528
Fayetteville, AR 72702
Fax: 501-521-9100
Phone: 501-521-4920
Web site: www.ozarkcoop.com
Serves AL, AK, FL, GA, KS, LA, MI, MS, OK, SC, TN, and TX

Tucson Cooperative Warehouse
350 S. Toole Ave
Tucson, AZ 85701
Fax: 520-792-3241
Phone: 800-350-2667

Web site: www.tcwfoodcoop.com
Serves AR, NM, West TX, Southern CA, Southern NV, UT, and
CO.

ORDER ORGANIC AND
NATURAL FOOD ON-LINE

A GROWING trend in buying organic and natural food is through
on-line services. Several national on-line supermarkets—including such as Walnut Acres, Whole Foods, and Wild Oats—deliver
a wide variety of vegetables, including meat and dairy to your
home through the mail. Although buying from national locations
like these has yet to become widespread, they offer an extensive
selection of organic foods, and it is a great way to buy otherwise
hard-to-find organic specialty foods and ingredients.

In addition, in several cities you can find delivery services that
for organic and natural foods including Atlanta, Seattle, and
Chicago. These services are able to provide fresh produce—mostly from local farmers—and often other food items as well such as
dairy and meat.

Here is a short list of places where you can buy organic produce
on-line—as well as local delivery services:

Walnut Acres
   Full line organic—from cereals to meats to vegetables. Many
      products sold directly from Walnut Acres organic farm—
      in operation for over fifty years.
   Phone: 1-800-344-9025
   Web site: www.walnutacres.com

MotherNature.Com
   Phone: 1-800-517-9020
   Web site: www.Mothernature.com

Offers dry goods such as vitamin, supplements, baby products, bath and beauty products, herbs, natural home supplies, coffee, tea and cleaning products.

Wild Oats Market
Phone: 303-440-5220 (home office in Boulder, CO)
Web site: www.wildoats.com
Full line natural grocery store.

Whole Foods Market (now Whole People)
Phone: 1-888-945-3637
Fax: 303-474-2700
Web site: www.wholefoods.org
Full line natural and organic grocery store.

Sunshine Organic Foods
PO Box 258
Watsonville, CA 95077
Phone: 831-728-9218
Web site: www.sunshineorganic.com
Complete selection of natural and conventional groceries— shop online for delivery in the San Diego Metro area.

Pioneer Organics
102 1/2 NW 36th
Seattle, WA 98107
Phone: 206-632-3424
Fax: 206-632-0609
Web site: www.pioneerorganics.com
Seattle area service—"The Puget Sound's premier organic produce home delivery service." Variety boxes delivered year-round with 100 percent certified organic produce. Weekly or every other week delivery available. Order online.

Urban Organic
   230A 7th Street
   Brooklyn, NY 11215
   Phone: 718-499-4321
   Fax: 718-499-3188
   Web site: www.urbanorganic.net
   Ships boxes of organic produce nationwide except for Alaska
      and Hawaii. In addition to fruit and vegetable boxes, also
      offers organic groceries, fresh-baked bread, soy products,
      herbs and spices, dairy products, desserts and more. Free
      shipping in most areas.

Planet Organics
   915 Cole St #172
   San Francisco, CA. 94117
   Phone: 1-800-956-5855 or 415-522-0526
   Fax: 415-648-2597
   Web site: www.planet-organics.com
   Home and office delivery of organic produce in San Francisco
      Bay area.

Green Grocer
   Washington, DC
   Phone: 202-789-2250
   Web site: www.washingtonsgreengrocer.com/indexx.html
   Delivery of farm fresh organic produce, including eggs and
      dairy.

Webvan.com
   310 Lakeside Dr
   Foster City, CA 94404
   Phone: 1-800-799-4999 (SF/Oakland area only)
   Web site: www.000103.webvan.com
   Currently, located only in the San Francisco/Oakland area
      (although it has building plans for distribution centers

near Chicago, Washington, Dallas, Seattle, Los Angeles, and more than 20 other markets across the country.) Webvan acts like a regular grocery store delivery system— with a special emphasis on locally grown produce. While Webvan has conventional brand name foods, it also has a solid selection of organic food available.

GROW YOUR OWN!

WHEN YOU decide to grow your own produce, the rewards go well beyond great food. While you probably can't grow all your food, you'd be surprised how many vegetables—both in numbers and variety—you can grow in most climates in the U.S. Growing food in your backyard can be especially enjoyable because it helps strengthen and diversify your own backyard ecosystem.

Organic gardeners usually start off by building up healthy, rich soil fed constantly with organic matter—such as material from your compost pile—including kitchen scraps, leaves and animal manure. Improved soil adds valuable nutrients, loosens clay-based soil, and improves drainage. Organic gardening also usually involves extensive mulching, crop rotation and often integrates herbs, flowers and vegetables. Certain flowers like marigolds, pansies and scented geraniums deter pests such as aphids, Japanese beetles, nematodes, snails, and slugs.

By not using toxic pesticides in your garden, you avoid killing bugs and beneficial insects like bees and ladybugs, ground beetles, lacewings, and spiders. There are several effective natural pest controls (such as milky spore for Japanese beetle grubs and Deer Off for deer). Many organic gardeners also employ homemade treatments such as soap spray for aphids, a mixture of yeast and sugar water for slugs, and hot-pepper spray for other pests. Or they may use "floating row cover," which is fabric, similar to cheesecloth, that covers plants and is porous to air, water, and sunlight, but not insects. An option of last resort is a bottle of Bt,

(Bacillus thuringiensis), the non-genetically engineered variety, of course, in organic spray form.

For tips, suggestions, and information on growing in your backyard, find an issue of the bible of organic gardening—*Organic Gardening Magazine.* Or see Maria Rodale's *Organic Gardening.* Information can be found at: www.organicgardening.com.

The Rodale Institute also has a plethora of information on organic gardening, including numerous books and articles, and a reference center for questions. For information on their books, give them a call at: 800-832-6285, or check out their website: www.rodaleinstitute.org.

Another excellent resource for gardeners is GardenWeb, which hosts a number of forums, including one on organic gardening. These forums help to answer questions, and acquire seeds and offer gardening tips. The website is: www.gardenweb.com.

See Chapter 10 for additional gardening resources.

COMMUNITY GARDENS

IF YOU live in a city and don't have your own yard or land to garden, look for a community garden. An estimated 10,000 community gardens now grace U.S. cities nationwide. Community gardens have the added benefit of bringing your community closer together.

For more information about how to start and run a community garden, check in with the American Community Gardening Association (ACGA)—a national, nonprofit membership organization of professionals, volunteers and supporters of community gardens in both urban and rural communities. The ACGA will soon have a searchable database on-line to locate community gardens nationwide. The ACGA also hosts a listserve that helps answer common questions surrounding community gardening.

Another group to check in with is the Urban Community Garden website. This website contains links very helpful to locating resources and community gardening organizations in your community: alexia.lis.uiuc.edu/~sewells/communitygardens.htm.

American Community Garden Network
100 N 20th Street, 5th Floor
Philadelphia, PA 19103-1495
Phone: 215-988-8785
Fax: 215-988-8810
Web site: www.communitygarden.org/index.html

ORGANIC SEEDS

WHEN GROWING your own food, make sure to buy organic or natural seeds, particularly traditional heirloom seeds, also known as open-pollinated or standard seeds. High quality seeds help to ensure biodiversity and protect the vibrancy of your garden. Organic seeds are the only seeds guaranteed to be GE-free.

Open-pollinated seeds propagate themselves by pollinating themselves or other plants. Pollination is carried out by wind, insects, or other natural carrying agents. During open-pollination, pollen is constantly being exchanged among dozens, or hundreds, and even thousands of plants that vary slightly genetically. The mixing of genetic material maintains the vibrancy of particular strains of plants, their ability to fight off disease and adapt to ever changing environmental conditions.

Heirloom or open-pollinating seeds are available through a number of natural seed companies. There are several options for purchasing these seeds both through the mail and over the internet. Ask your seed source whether their seeds are genetically engineered—particularly if you are growing potatoes, or sweet corn. (See chapter 10 for a list of companies using organic seeds.)

One of the largest organic seed companies is Seeds of Change (www.seedsofchange.com) 1–888–762–7333. They sell 100 percent non-genetically engineered seeds. Seed Savers Exchange is another seed source dedicated to helping backyard farmers retain the genetic diversity of seeds and grow non-GE vegetables and other plants. The exchange describes a number of seed varieties with traits developed outside of genetic engineering. See chapter 10 for additional seed companies which have organic or natural seeds.

Johnny's Selected Seeds in Maine (www.johnnyseeds.com) is one of eight companies in New England, and forty in the U.S. and Canada, to sign onto the Safe Seed Initiative, a project launched by heirloom seed grower Tom Stearns (High Mowing Organic Seeds, Wolcott, Vermont, 802-888-1800) with the assistance of Vermont-NOFA (Northeast Organic Farming Association) (www.nofavt.org) and the Boston-based Council for Responsible Genetics (www.gene-watch.org). See chapter 7, for list of companies that have signed the pledge.

RESTAURANTS

A GROWING number of chefs nationwide are striving to buy and serve locally and organically produced foods. In fact, several hundred of the nation's top chefs advocate avoiding GE foods and ingredients and using organic ingredients whenever possible. Some of these top chefs include: Alice Waters (Chez Panisse Café and Restaurant, Café Fanny, Berkeley, CA), Nora Pouillon (Restaurant Noras, Washington, DC), Rick Bayless (Topolobampo and Frontera Grill, Chicago), Jesse Cool (Flea Street Cafe, Menlo Park, CA), Stan Frankenthaler (Salamander Restaurant, Cambridge), Peter Hoffman (Savoy, New York), Lucia Watson (Lucias Restaurant and Wine Bar, Minneapolis), and Charlie Trotter (Charlie Trotters, Chicago).

Many of these top chefs leading this new wave of cooking are a part of the nationwide network called the Chefs Collaborative. The Chefs Collaborative (www.chefnet.com/cc2000) has over 1,500 chefs nationwide helping to promote sustainable cuisine by teaching children, supporting local farmers, educating one another, and inspiring the public to choose good, clean food.

The Chefs Collaborative works to improve recycling in kitchens, donating food to the hungry, buying locally, and buying organic food. Chefs Collaborative is now working closely with schools on an education program that teaches children where their food comes from, and how it is prepared. The Adopt-A-School Program introduces kids to ways to eat healthy and protect their planet, and it incorporates the foods, culture, geography, and history of eight world regions (one of which is their own local region).

Chefs Collaborative has come out publicly in calling for the labeling of genetically engineered foods.[11]

Many of the nation's top chefs are going beyond simply trying to use organic ingredients, and are actively quizzing their suppliers on genetically engineered ingredients. Alice Waters, of Chez Panisse, has told her suppliers that her restaurant will be GE-free by the end of 2000. At Seattle's Dahlia Lounge, chef Matt Costello has eliminated most genetically modified ingredients and is moving toward a total ban. In Philadelphia, the White Dog Cafe is also working toward a total ban. In April 2000, nearly 30 chefs in Philadelphia held a press conference denouncing the new technology and demanding labeling.

Among restaurateurs, Nora Pouillon has followed the emerging emphasis on organic most thoroughly. Her Washington, D.C. restaurant, Restaurant Nora, is the only in the country to be certified organic—95 percent of her ingredients are organic. Others in the industry are taking notice: Pouillon won the "Award of Excellence" in the "Chef of the Year" category at the annual International Association for Culinary Professionals 1997 Awards Ceremony.

These leading chefs are not alone in their search for organic food and ingredients. In *Food & Wine* magazine's 1997 Chef's Survey, 76 percent of those chefs surveyed responded "Yes" to the question, "Do you actively seek out organically grown ingredients?"

HOW YOU CAN SHOP
AND ACT WITH PURPOSE

GENETICALLY ENGINEERED food has slipped into our kitchens, lunchrooms and restaurants quietly—without the knowledge of most consumers. It is unlikely this new technology will leave our shelves in the same quiet manner. It is up to us to let food companies, supermarkets and the biotech industry know that we don't want these "novel" foods. It will take an informed and concerted consumer action—both at home and in the body politic—to pressure U.S. regulatory agencies to become more vigilant. And we need to demand that our elected representatives put forth a policy on genetically engineered foods that ensures the food supply is safe and that gives consumers all pertinent information about exactly what we are eating.

SHOPPING WITH PURPOSE

AS A food consumer, every dollar you spend on food not only has practical value helping to feed you and your family, but also delivers a political and economic message about what kind of agricultural system you support. In effect, you vote every time you buy food. Every dollar you spend on processed food, junk food, or genetically engineered food sends one message. But every dollar you spend on organic or natural food, locally grown food, or on food grown outside of the supermarket system (farmers markets, CSA's, co-ops, etc.), sends another message—that you want food to be safe, fresh and environmentally-friendly. As we've already discussed, the food industry is slowly starting to "get it" and is introducing a wide array of organic food products. But it is up to all of us to push the industry further by spending our consumer dollars responsibly.

Aside from trying to avoid purchasing genetically engineered foods, there are several other small but significant steps you can take at your grocery store. The most effective way to influence your local grocer or a particular food company is to write a letter directly to its corporate headquarters. While letters or faxes take time to write, they hold the greatest weight among companies. Companies are obligated to respond—and if you ask them specific questions, it is more difficult for them to respond with a form letter. Ask the companies whether they sell genetically engineered foods, how they identify which foods contain genetically engineered ingredients, and demand that they make more information available for consumers. You can also call them on the telephone on their toll-free "consumer comment" lines and request that they put their policies on genetically engineered foods in writing. A list of America's 25 major food companies and contact information is available in chapter 6 and the Organic Consumer Association has posted a list of the phone numbers of the Frankenfoods 15, leading American food companies that have refused to guarantee that their foods are GE-free on the internet at www.purefood.org.

WHILE COMMON sense tells us that the food we feed our children should be the safest and most nutritious available, a trip to the school lunchroom often tells a different story. In fact, most schools offer more junk food than ever—soft drinks, candy bars, and a wide variety of processed, packaged food. This growing menu of generally unhealthy food is increasing at shocking rates nationwide.

It is important to remember that your tax dollars support your schools. Local school boards offer an opportunity to affect what the children of your community are fed each day for lunch. In every part of the country, there are opportunities to limit exposures to genetically engineered food by following the recommendations outlined in this book.

Changes are beginning to take place. The school district in Berkeley, California has already acted to dramatically change its school lunch program. After concerned parents visited school officials regarding the district's school lunch program, Berkeley schools developed a lunch program that bans the use of genetically engineered foods, irradiated foods, and dairy products from cows injected with the recombinant Bovine Growth Hormone (rBGH). Other goals of the district's plan include establishing a child nutrition advisory committee and eliminating food additives and high-fat, high-sugar snacks and entrees.

In addition, over the next several years, Berkeley will offer organic food for lunch. Administrators hope to defray some of the added expense of purchasing organic foods by growing 25 percent of the produce on the campuses themselves. Eleven of Berkeley's 16 schools already have gardens. Also in California, Santa Monica schools have experimented with a Farmers Market salad bar. More information on the Berkeley program can be found at: www.foodsystems.com. Similar programs to push organic, and decrease the use of genetically engineered ingredients, are being considered at a number of schools and universities around the country.

LEGISLATING TO PROTECT CONSUMERS

MOST U.S. legislators know very little about genetically engineered foods and their potential threats to human health and the environment. It is absolutely critical that we let our legislators know of our concerns about the environmental and human health threats of genetically engineered foods and the lack of available pertinent information for consumers about these foods.

The biotech and food industry have spent large amounts of money in campaign contributions to influence legislators on this issue. According to an analysis done in November 1999 by the Center for Responsive Politics, members of the Alliance for Better Foods (a trade group set up to advocate for biotechnology) during the first nine months of 1999, gave more than $676,000 in soft money, PAC and individual contributions to members of Congress—83 percent to Republicans. In addition, biotech giants Monsanto, DuPont and Novartis Seeds, spent more than $6 million lobbying members of Congress and the Clinton administration in 1998.

Contacting your U.S. congressperson or state representatives is not difficult. In fact, most legislators want to hear from their constituents. Once again, letter writing is the best way to communicate your concerns. Each letter sent to a legislator is counted and tracked. Of course, phone calls and even e-mails are also effective ways to communicate with your legislator. If you have time, it is always worthwhile to set up meeting with your representative or their staff to discuss your concerns.

As we discuss in chapter 5, a number of innovative legislative measures are being introduced to address genetically engineered foods, at the national, state, and local levels. Find out where your state and federal legislators stand on these issues and urge them to take action if they haven't already.

THE FOOD and Drug Administration (what we eat), the Environmental Protection Agency (the environment) and the U.S. Department of Agriculture (what we grow) regulate genetically engineered foods (For more details, see chapter 5). As Federal entities, they operate under the President and the cabinet secretaries he appoints. It is important that consumers let those at regulatory agencies and the President know that GE crops are not adequately regulated and that immediate steps need to be taken to ensure the safety of human health and the environment.

All three regulatory agencies routinely engage in what is called the "rule-making" process, and frequently ask for public input on a number of agency policies. The websites of all three agencies (www.fda.gov, www.epa.gov, www.usda.gov) provide timely information, and opportunities for public comment. Keep an eye out for opportunities to submit your own comments to these agencies regarding their policies on genetically engineered foods and other food and agriculture issues. Public comments can have a big impact at agencies. For instance, when the USDA proposed national organic rules that were riddled with harmful loopholes, nearly 300,000 citizens submitted comments. The agency scrapped the first proposed rules and re-wrote them—paying special attention to citizens' comments.

ORGANIZATIONS AND CAMPAIGNS

IF YOU'RE ready to become more active on the issue of genetic engineering, there are a number of organizations and campaigns that could use your help. A great way to get plugged in is to join one of the following groups and their campaigns:

- Friends of the Earth (FOE)—Friends of the Earth's Safer Food, Safer Farm campaign is targeting U.S. federal agencies to better regulate of GE foods and crops. FOE has called for a moratorium on further releases into the environment of all GE crops. FOE is organizing demonstrations outside major supermarket chains, calling on the stores to remove all GE ingredients from their own brand label. FOE is also working with shareholders to hold food and biotech corporations accountable. For more information on FoE's Safer Food, Safer Farms campaign, visit their website at: www.foe.org/safefood.

- Greenpeace USA—Greenpeace has been a leading opponent worldwide to genetically engineered foods. In the U.S., Greenpeace has sued the EPA regarding the environmental impacts of genetically engineered crops, successfully convinced Gerber baby foods to go GE-free, and targeted a number of other U.S. food companies through protests and other actions. Greenpeace is organizing a "True Food Network" to fight genetically engineered food. To join the network, call 1–800–326–0959, or go to: www.greenpeaceusa.org/ge.

- Organic Consumers Association—The OCA organizes within food co-ops and among consumers of organic food in all 50 states. OCA has helped organize consumers to submit comments to federal agencies, and directly target food companies that use genetically engineered ingredients. OCA is currently targeting what it calls, "The Frankenfoods 15" food companies that are using this technology. For more information, call 218–726–1443, or go to: www.purefood.org.

- Foundation on Economic Trends—Run by long-time biotech opponent, Jeremy Rifkin, this organization recently organized a massive lawsuit against Monsanto and other biotech companies, charging that they were violating U.S. anti-trust laws. This vital lawsuit directly challenges the biotech industry and their attempt to control all aspects of agriculture. For more information, visit www.biotechcentury.org.

- Center for Food Safety—The Center is a non-profit legal firm in Washington, D.C. which has filed two ground-breaking lawsuits against U.S. regulatory agencies. The first challenges the FDA's policy on genetically engineered foods, demanding that the agency require safety testing and labeling of these novel foods. The second challenges the EPA's regulation of genetically engineered Bt crops—calling for the agency to conduct more thorough analysis of risks before the products enter the market. For more information go to: www.centerforfoodsafety.org. (For an additional listing of organizations, websites, and other information resources, see chapter 10.)

10

WHERE TO FIND OUT MORE

OTHER BOOKS ON GENETIC ENGINEERING

Fox, Michael, *Eating with Conscience: The Bioethics of Food* (NewSage Press, 1997).

Ho, Mae-Wan, *Genetic Engineering: Dream or Nightmare* (Gateway Books, 1998).

Jack, Alex, *Imagine a World Without Monarch Butterflies* (One Peaceful World Press, 1999).

Kimbrell, Andrew, *The Human Body Shop: The Engineering and Marketing of Life* (Harper Collins, 1993).

Kneen, Brewster, *Farmageddon:Food and the Culture of Biotechnology*, (New Society Publishers, 1999).

Lappe, Mark and Britt Baily, *Against the Grain* (Common Courage Press, 1998).

Nottingham, S, *Eat Your Genes: How Genetically Modified Food Is Entering Our Diet*, (Zed Books, 1998).

Rifkin, Jeremy, *The Biotech Century* (Tarcher/Putnam, 1998).

Shiva, Vandana, *Biopiracy: The Plunder of Nature and Knowledge* (South End Press, 1997).

Teitel, Martin and Kimberly A. Wilson, *Genetically Engineered Food: Changing the Nature of Nature*, (Park Street Press, 1999).

Ticciati, Laura and Robin Ticcati, *Genetically Engineered Foods: Are They Safe? You Decide* (Keats, 1998).

Turney, Jon. *Frankenstein's Footsteps: Science, Genetics and Popular Culture* (Yale University Press, 1998).

ORGANIZATIONS AND WEBSITES

Genetically Engineered Foods

National

Alliance for Bio-Integrity
406 W Depot Ave
Fairfield, IA 52556
Phone: 515-472-5554
Web site: www.bio-integrity.org

BioDemocracy Campaign
6114 Highway 61
Little Marais, MN 55614
Phone: 218-226-4164
Web site: www.purefood.org

Bioengineering Action Network of North America
Web site: www.tao.ca/~ban/

Campaign to Label Genetically Engineered Foods
PO Box 55699
Seattle, WA 98155
Phone: 425-771-4049
Web site: www.thecampaign.org

Center for Ethics and Toxics
39141 S Highway 1
PO Box 673
Gualala, CA 95445
Phone: 707-884-1700
Website: www.cetos.org

Center for Food Safety
66 Pensylvania Ave SE Suite#302
Washington, DC 20003
Phone: 202-547-9359
Web site: www.centerforfoodsafety.org

Chefs Collaborative
www.chefnet.com/cc2000

Citizens for Health
Phone: 800-357-2211
Web site: www.citizens.org

Consumers Union
101 Truman Ave
Yonkers, NY 10703
Phone: 914-378-2452
Web site: www.consumersunion.org/food/food.htm

Council for Responsible Genetics
5 Upland Road, Suite 3
Cambridge, MA 02140
Phone: 617-868-0870
Web site: www.gene-watch.org

The Edmonds Institute
20319 92nd Avenue West
Edmonds, WA 98020
Phone: 425-775-5383
Web site: www.edmonds-institute.org

Environmental Defense
257 Park Avenue South
New York, NY 10010
Phone: 800-684-3322
Web site: www.edf.org

Foundation on Economic Trends
1660 L Street NW, Suite 216
Washington DC 20036
Phone: 202-466-2823
Web site: www.biotechcentury.org

Friends of the Earth
1025 Vermont Ave NW
Washington, DC 20005-6303
Phone: 202-783-7400, 877-843-8687
Fax: 202-783-0444
Web site: www.foe.org

Institute for Agriculture and Trade Policy
2105 1st Avenue South

Minneapolis, MN 55404
Phone: 612-870-0453
Web site: www.iatp.org

Greenpeace USA
564 Mission Street
PO Box 416
San Francisco, CA 94105
Phone: 1-800-326-0959
Web site: www.greenpeaceusa.org/ge/

Mothers and Others for a Livable Planet
40 West 20th Street
New York, NY 10011-4211
Phone: 212-242-0010
Web site: www.igc.apc.org/mothers/

Mothers for Natural Law
PO Box 1900
Fairfield, IA 52556
515-472-2040
Web site: www.safe-food.org

People's Earth Network
2192 Massachusetts Ave
Cambridge, MA 02140
Phone: 617-491-7646
Web site: www.peoplesearth.org

Rural Advancement Foundation International
PO Box 640
Pittsboro, NC 27312
Phone: 919-542-1396
Web site: www.rafi.org

Union of Concerned Scientists
2 Brattle Square
Cambridge, MA 02238-9105
Phone: 617-547-5552
Web site: www.ucsusa.org

Regional/Local
Northeast Resistance Against Genetic Engineering
Vermont Clearinghouse
c/o Institute for Social Ecology
1118 Maple Hill Rd

Plainfield, VT 05667
Phone: 802-454-9957
Web site: www.bckweb.com/nerage/

NW RAGE
P.O. Box 15289
Portland, OR 97293
Phone: 503-236-5772 ext. 2
Web site: www.nwrage.org/nwrage.html

Gateway Greens
P.O. Box 8094
St. Louis, MO 63156
Phone: 314-771-8576
Web site: www.greens.org/s-r/gga/

Rural Vermont
15 Barre Street
Montpelier, VT 05602
Phone: 802-223-7222
Web site: www.greenfornewengland.org/members/rural.html

International
Institute of Science in Society (ISIS)
Web site: www.i-sis.dircon.co.uk

Physicians and Scientists for Responsible Application of Science and Technology
(PSRAST)
Web site: www.pcrm.org

Third World Network
Web site: www.twnside.org.sg

Pesticides

Pesticide Action Network of North America
49 Powell St, Suite 500
San Francisco, CA 94102
Phone: 415-981-1771
Web site: www.panna.org

National Coalition Against the Misuse of Pesticides
701 E Street, SE, Suite 200
Washington, DC 20003

Phone: 202-543-5450
Web site: www.ncamp.org

Organic

Committee for Sustainable Agriculture
406 Main St #313
Watsonville, CA 95076
Phone: 831-763-2111
Web site: www.csa-efc.org

Community Alliance with Family Farmers CA
PO Box 363
Davis, CA 95617
Phone: 530-756-8518
Web site: www.caff.org

Henry Wallace Institute for Alternative Agriculture at Winrock International
9200 Edmonston Rd, Suite 117
Greenbelt, MD 20770-1551
Phone: 301-441-8777.
Fax: 301-220-0164
Web site: www.hawiaa.org/hawiaa.htm

Organic Alliance
400 Selby Ave, Suite T
St. Paul, MN 55102
Phone: 651-265-3678
Web site: www.organic.org

Organic Consumers Association
6114 Highway 61
Little Marais, MN 55614
Phone: 218-726-1443
Web site: www.purefood.org

Organic Farm Research Foundation
P.O. Box 440
Santa Cruz, CA 95061
Phone: 831-426-6606
Web site: www.ofrf.org

Organic Materials Review Institute
Box 11558
Eugene, OR 97440-3758

Phone: 541-343-7600
Web site: www.omri.org

Organic Trade Association
  74 Fairview St
  PO Box 547
  Greenfield, MA 01302
  Phone: 413-774-7511
  Web site: www.ota.com

Organic Farmers Marketing Association
  8364 S SR 39
  Clayton, IN 46118
  Web site: web.iquest.net/ofma/

Rodale Institute
  611 Siegfriedale Rd
  Kutztown, PA 19530
  Phone: 610-683-1400 (experimental farm), 800-832-6285 (bookstore)
  Web site: www.rodaleinstitute.org

USDA National Organic Program
  Web site: www.ams.usda.gov/nop

Community Supported Agriculture Programs

Sustainable Agriculture Network
  www.sare.org/san/csa/index.htm

USDA Alternative Farming Systems Information Center
  www.nal.usda.gov/afsic/csa/

CSA's By State
  www.umass.edu/umext/csa

Farmer's Market Online
  www.farmersmarketonline.com/Communit.htm

Center for Agroecology & Sustainable Food Systems
  University of California, Santa Cruz
  zzyx.ucsc.edu/casfs/index

Community Supported Agriculture in Maine
  www.state.me.us./agriculture/marketprod/communityag.htm

Farmers' Markets

Community Support (resource page)
Web site: www.farmersmarketonline.com/Communit.htm

Farmer's Markets
Web site: www.farmersmarketonline.com/index.html

USDA's Farmer's Market Source
Web site: www.ams.usda.gov/farmersmarkets/

Missouri Alternatives Center
agebb.missouri.edu/mac/

New Mexico Farmers Marketing Association
Web site: www.farmersmarketsnm.org

The Small Farm Program USDA-Cooperative
State Research, Education and Extension Service
Web site: www.reeusda.gov/smallfarm

Sustainable Agriculture Network
Web site: www.sare.org

Urban Agriculture Notes/City Farmer
Canada's Office of Urban Agriculture
Web site: www.cityfarmer.org

USDA Agricultural Marketing Service
Farmer Direct Marketing
Farm Direct Marketing Bibliography, Part 8.
www.ams.usda.gov/directmarketing/b_8.htm

Community Gardening

American Community Garden Network
100 N 20th St, 5th Floor
Philadelphia, PA 19103-1495
Phone: 215-988-8785
Fax: 215-988-8810
Web site: www.communitygarden.org/index.html

Co-ops

U.S. Food Co-op Directory
  Web site: www.purefood.org/coopindex.htm

Co-op Network
  Box 57
  Randolph, VT 05060
  Phone: 802-234-9293
  Web site: http:/users.quest-net.com/~george.keller/index.html

Center for Cooperatives
  University of California
  One Shields Ave,
  Davis, CA 95616
  Phone: 530-752-2408
  Web site: www.cooperatives.ucdavis.edu

Cooperative Development Institute
  277 Federal St
  Greenfield, MA 01301
  Phone: 413-774-7599

Cooperative Development Services
  30 West Mifflin St, Suite 401
  Madison, WI 53703
  Phone: 608-258-4396

Organic and Natural Seed Companies

Farmers Market Online
  Web site: www.FarmersMarketOnline.com/index.html

Abundant Life Seed Foundation
  P.O. Box 772
  930 Lawrence St
  Port Townsend, WA 98368
  Phone: 206-385-5660
  Web site: www.csf.colorado.edu/perma/abundant/
  E-mail: abundant@olypen.com

Bountiful Gardens
  18001 Shafer Ranch Rd
  Willits, CA 95490-9626
  Phone: 707-459-6410
  Web site: www.bountifulgardens.com

E-mail: bountiful@zapcom.net
Rare grains, herbs, compost crops, and European heirlooms. Affiliated with
   Ecology Action.

Burpee Heirloom Seed Catalog
   W. Atlee Burpee Co.
   300 Park Ave
   Warminister, PA 18991-0008
   Phone: 800-999-8552
   Web site: www.burpee.com
   Untreated seed upon request (except corn).

Butterbrooke Farm
   78 Barry Rd
   Oxford, CT 06483
   Phone: 203-888-2000
   Non-hybrid hardy vegetable strains raised by cooperating farmers. SASE for
      pricelist.

Comstock Ferre
   263 Main St
   Wethersfield, CT 06109
   Phone: 860-571-6590
   Web site: www.tiac.net/users/comstock
   E-mail: canstock@tiac.net

The Cook's Garden
   P.O. Box 535
   Londonderry, VT 05148
   Phone: 800-457-9713
   Web site: www.cooksgarden.com
   E-mail: orders@cooksgarden.com

Dacha Barinka
   46232 Strathcona Rd
   Chilliwack, BC V2P 3T2
   Phone: 604-792-0957

Down on the Farm Seeds
   P.O. Box 184
   Hiram, OH 44234
   Seedlist $1.00. Untreated heirloom/open-pollinated seed. By mail only.

Ed Hume Seeds, Inc.
   P.O. Box 1450
   Kent, WA 98035

Phone: 253-859-1110
Web site: www.humeseeds.com
E-mail: humeseeds@aol.com

Elixir Farm Botanicals
  General Delivery
  Brixey, MO 65618
  Contact: Lavinia McKinney
  Phone: 417-261-2393
  Web site: www.elixirfarm.com
  E-mail: efb@aristotle.net
  Biodynamically certified organic seed of native and Chinese medicinal herbs.

FEDCO Seeds
  P.O. Box 520
  Waterville, ME 04903
  Phone: 207-873-7333
  Seed cooperative (website is private—customers only). $2.00 for catalog.

Fox Hollow Seed Co.
  P.O. Box 148
  McGrann, PA 16236
  Phone: 724-548-7333

Fruited Plain Seeds
  P.O. Box 56
  Craigville, IN 46731
  Phone: 219-565-3212
  E-mail: smz@adamswells.com
  Mostly cover crops. Also cleaning of food-grade seed for the organic industry.

Garden City Seeds
  778 Hwy 93 N
  Hamilton, MT 59840
  Phone: 406-961-4837
  E-mail: seeds@montana.com
  Trials and tests all Garden City vegetable varieties before offering for flavor, quick
    maturity, and vigor in the Far North. All seed is untreated, some organic.

Harris Seeds
  60 Saginaw Dr
  Rochester, NY 14692-2960
  Phone: 800-514-4441
  Web site: www.harrisseeds.com
  Offers some varieties untreated.

Heirloom Seeds
    PO Box 245
    West Elizabeth, PA 15088-0245
    Phone: 412-384-0852
    Web site: www.heirloomseeds.com
    E-mail: mail@heirloomseeds.com

Horizon Herbs
    P.O. Box 69
    Williams, OR 97544
    Phone: 541-846-6704
    Fax: 541-846-6233
    Web site: www.chatlink.com/~herbseed/
    E-mail: herbseed@chatlink.com

J.L. Hudson, Seedsman
    P.O. Box 1058
    Redwood City, CA 94064

Johnny's Selected Seeds
    Foss Hill Road
    Albion, ME 04910
    Phone: 207-437-9294
    Web site: www.johnnyseeds.com
    E-mail: johnnys@johnnyseeds.com
    Treated (T) or Untreated (U) indicated. Medicinal herb section.

The KUSA Society
    PO Box 761
    Ojai, CA 93024

Landis Valley Museum
    Heirloom Seed Project
    2451 Kissel Hill Rd
    Lancaster, PA 17601
    Phone:717-569-0401
    Web site: www.landisvalleymuseum.org
    Single packets of heirloom varieties of the Pennsylvania Dutch.

Ledden Brothers, Inc.
    PO Box 7
    195 Center Ave
    Sewell, NJ 08080-0007
    Phone: 888-783-7337
    Web site: www.leddens.com

E-mail: seeds@leddens.com
Untreated seed upon request.

Mighty Seed™
 Seed International, Inc.
 3208 Sue Circle
 Rio Rancho, NM 87124
 Phone: 505-892-7373 (request catalog)
 Web site: www.choicemall.com/mightyseed/
 E-mail: jckf777@aol.com
 Garden seeds for sprouting; grains for human and animal consumption,
  kosher seeds, grains and bean varieties, and un-treated and certified.

Moose Tubers
 PO Box 510
 Waterville, ME 04903
 Contact: Allison Lacourse
 Division of FEDCO—see above.

Native Seeds/SEARCH
 526 N. 4th Ave
 Tucson, AZ 85705-8450
 Phone: 520-622-5561 (no phone orders)
 Fax: 520-622-5591 (fax orders welcome)
 Web site: www.azstarnet.com/~nss
 E-mail: nss@az.starnet.com
 Native and traditional seeds of the Southwest. Nonprofit organization.
  Newsletter and publications.

The Natural Gardening Co.
 PO Box 750776
 Petaluma, CA 94975-0776
 Phone: 707-766-9303
 www.naturalgardening.com
 E-mail: info@naturalgardening.com
 Organically grown tomato seedlings and seeds of heirloom varieties.

Old Sturbridge Village Museum and Select Seeds
 1 Old Sturbridge Village Rd
 Sturbridge, MA 01566
 Phone: 508-347-3362
 Web site: www.oldsturbridgevillage.org
 E-mail: osvvc@osv.org

Peace Seeds
PO Box 190
Gila, NM 88038
Jointly publishes Deep Diversity Catalog with Seeds of Change.

Plants of the Southwest
Agua Fria Road, Route 6, Box 11A
Santa Fe, NM 87505
Phone: 800-788-7333
Web site: www.plantsofthesouthwest.com
E-mail: contact@pots.com
Web site features 130 native wildflowers. Also herbs, vegetables.

Pinetree Garden Seeds
PO Box 300
New Gloucester, ME 04260
Phone: 207-926-3400
Web site: www.superseeds.com
E-mail: superseeds@worldnet.att.net

Redwood City Seed Co.
PO Box 361
Redwood City, CA 94064
Phone: 650-325-7333
Web site: www.batnet.com/rwc-seed/index.html
Native seeds, open-pollinated vegetables. Pamphlets.

Ronniger's Seed Potatoes
PO Box 307
Ellensburg, WA 98926
Phone: 800-846-6178
Large selection of organically grown seed potatoes.

Seeds Blüm
27 Idaho City Stage Rd
Boise, ID 83716
Phone: 800-742-1423
(800) 528-3658 (to place an order)
Web site: www.seedsblum.com
E-mail: 103374.167@compuserve.com

Seeds of Change
PO Box 15700
Santa Fe, NM 87506
Phone: 888-762-7333
Web site: www.seedsofchange.com

Seeds of Diversity Canada
   Box 36 Stn Q
   Toronto, Ontario, M4T 2L7
   Phone: Tel: 905-623-0353
   Web site: www.seeds.ca or e-mail at mail@seeds.ca.
   E-mail: mail@seeds.ca

Seed Dreams
   PO Box 1476
   Santa Cruz, CA 95061-1476
   E-mail: sr012@csufresno.edu
   Old-time heirloom vegetable and grain seeds, open-pollinated and organic.
      Will donate seeds to any children's gardening project.

Seed Savers Exchange
   3076 North Winn Road
   Decorah, IA 52101
   Phone: (319) 382-5990
   All packets heirloom seed, $2.50/pkt.
   Web site: www.seedsavers.org

Seed Savers Garden Store
   1919 Monroe Street
   Madison, WI 53711
   Phone: 608-280-8149
   Website: www.seedsavers.org/wholepgs/mainpgs/Madisonstore/htm

Seeds West Garden Seeds
   317 14th Street NW
   Albuquerque, NM 87104
   Phone: 505-843-9713
   Web site: www.seedswestgardenseeds.com
   E-mail: seeds@nmia.com
   Heirloom garden seed for the Southwest. New owners 1998.

Southern Exposure Seed Exchange
   PO Box 460
   Mineral, VA 23117
   Phone: 540-894-9480
   Web site: www.southernexposure.com
   E-mail: gardens@southernexposure.com
   Catalog $2.00. Heirloom/open-pollinated seeds, alliums, fruit trees.

Stokes Seeds
   PO Box 548
   Buffalo, NY 14240-0548

Phone: 716-695-6980
Web site: www.stokeseeds.com
E-mail: stokes@stokeseeds.com
U.S. office of Canadian company; large selection, bulk (catalog not online).

Territorial Seed Company
PO Box 157
Cottage Grove, OR 97424-0061
Phone: 888-657-3131
Web site: www.territorial-seed.com
E-mail: tetrl@srvl.vsite.com

Thomas Jefferson Center for Historic Plants, Monticello
PO Box 318
Charlottesville, VA 22902.

Thompson & Morgan
PO Box 1308
Jackson, NJ 08527-0308
Phone: 800-274-7333
Web site: www.thompson-morgan.com
E-mail: tminc@thompson-morgan.com
Large selection ornamental, vegetables.

Tomato Growers Supply Co.
PO Box 2237
Fort Myers, FL 33902
Phone: 941-768-1119 (Customer Service),
    888-478-7333 (orders)
Fax: 888-768-3476
Web site: www.tomatogrowers.com
Heirloom tomatoes; most varieties untreated.

The Tomato Seed Co., Inc.
PO Box 323
Metuchen, NJ 08840
Phone: (201) 548-9036
Heirloom tomatoes.

Turtle Enterprises
Route 1, Box 71
Dalton, WI 53926
SASE for catalog of sweet sorghum varieties.

Shepard's Garden Seeds
   30 Irene St.
   Torrington,CT 06790-0658
   Phone: 860-482-3638
   Web site: www.shepherdseeds.com
   E-mail: custsrv@shepherdseeds.com

William Dam Seeds
   PO Box 8400
   279 Hwy 8 (West Flamboro)
   Dundas, Ontario L9H 6M1,Canada
   Phone: 905-628-6641
   E-mail: willdam@sympatico.ca
   European, Oriental vegetables and houseplant seeds.

Organic Garden Fertilizer Sources

Garden Supplies:
Gardens Alive
   5100 Schenley Place
   Lawrenceburg, IN 47025
   Phone: 812-537-8651 (Customer Service)
   Web site: www.gardens-alive.com
   Offers high quality lawn and garden products that work with nature.

Planet Natural
   1612 Gold Ave.
   PO Box 3146
   Bozeman, MT 59772
   Phone: 406-587-5891 (Information), 800-289-6656 (Orders)
   Web site: www.planetnatural.com
   E-mail: ecostore@mcn.net
   Catalogue sales, specializing in natural pest controls.

Nitron Industries
   PO Box 1447
   Fayetteville, AR 72702
   Phone: 800-835-0123
   Web site: www.nitron.com
   Nitron Industries is the premier source for organic fertilizers, soil amend-
       ments, non-hybrid seeds, and insect controls for lawns, gardens, and
       flower beds.

Bio-Organics Home Gardener Center
   3200 Corte Malpaso, #107
   Camarillo, CA 93102

Phone: 800-604-0444
Fax: 805-389-3773
Web site: www.chappyspowerorganics.com

Peaceful Valley
PO Box 2209
Grass Valley, CA 95945
Phone: 530-272-4769
Web site: www.groworganic.com
E-mail: contact@groworganic.com
Primarily mail-order catalogue sales. Great diversity of offerings. Consulting
    service.

Bountiful Gardens
18001 Shafer Ranch Rd
Willits, CA 95490-9626
Phone: 707-459-6410
Web site: www.bountifulgardens.com
E-mail: bountiful@zapcom.net
Catalogue sales, specializing in seed. Focus on biointensive farming and gar-
    dening. Good source for small quantities of hard-to-find covercrop seed.

Harmony Farm Supply & Nursery
3244 Gravenstein Hwy N.
Sebastopol, CA 95472
Phone: 707-823-9125
E-mail: info@harmonyfarm.com
Web site: www.harmonyfarm.com
Primarily mail-order catalogue sales. Great diversity of offerings. Current cat-
    alogue: $2.00.

Ledden Brothers, Inc.
195 Center Ave.
PO Box 7
Sewell, NJ 08080-0007
Phone: 888-783-7337
Web site: www.leddens.com
E-mail: seeds@leddens.com
Primarily mail-order catalogue and retail sales. Emphasis on seed and garden
    supplies.

Organic Growers Supply
PO Box 520
Waterville, ME 04903
Phone: 207-873-7333
Primarily mail-order catalogue sales.

The Invisible Gardener
  PO Box 4311
  Malibu, CA 90265
  Phone: 310-457-4438
  Web site: www.invisiblegardener.com
  For natural pest control and more.

Organic/Natural Meat

Alaska Natural Beef
  Bering Pacific Ranch
  Umnak Island
  Box 326
  Unalaska, AK 99685
  Phone: 888-384-5366
  Web site: www.alaskanatural.com
  E-mail: okmok@alaskanatural.com

Coleman Natural Products Inc.
  5140 Race Court
  Denver, CO 80216
  Web site: www.colemanmeats.com
  Phone: 303-297-9393
  E-mail: coleman@colemannatural.com
  Available in many national grocery stores and coops. Find retail location clos-
  est to you on their Web site.

Laura's Lean Beef
  2285 Executive Drive, Suite 200
  Lexington, KY 40505
  Phone: 606-299-7707, 800-487-5326
  Web site: www.laurasleanbeef.com
  E-mail: llb@laurasleanbeef.com

Organic Valley Family of Farms
  CROPP Cooperative
  507 W. Main Street
  La Farge, WI 54639
  Phone: 888-444-6455
  Web site: www.organicvalley.com
  E-mail: organic@organicvalley.com

Miscellaneous

Seven Bridges Cooperative
  419 May Avenue

Santa Cruz, CA 95060
800-769-4409
Web site: www.breworganic.com
E-mail: 7bridges@breworganic.com
Organic beer brewing ingredients and supplies.

Government

U.S. Department of Agriculture
www.aphis.usda.gov/biotechnology/

U.S. Environmental Protection Agency
www.epa.gov/pesticides/biopesticides/

U.S. Food and Drug Administration
www.fda.gov/oc/biotech/default.htm

U.S. House of Representatives
www.house.gov

U.S. Senate
www.senate.gov

ENDNOTES

INTRODUCTION

1. For a summary of U.S. and international consumer polls on genetically engineered foods see the Web site of the Consumers International: <www.consumersinternational.org/campaigns/biotech/surveys.html>
2. Marian Burros, "Biotechnology's Bounty," *New York Times* (May 21,1997) and Marian Burros, "Eating Well: Genes are Changed, but Not the Label," *New York Times* (September 8, 1999).
3. Mike Hendricks, "Labels Not Required to Reveal All," *Kansas City Star* (March 7, 1994).

CHAPTER 1

1. Hord, Bill, "Farmers Warned of Uncertainties With Crops Genetics," *Omaha World-Herald* (March 4, 2000).

2. Hansen, Michael, "Genetic Engineering Is Not An Extension of Conventional Plant Breeding," Consumer Policy Institute (January 27, 2000). Submitted to the Food and Drug Administration.

3. Kimbrell, Andrew, *The Human Body Shop: The Engineering and Making of Life*, (HarperCollins, 1993) p. 176.

4. Bergelson, J., Purrington, CB and G. Wichmann. 1998. "Promiscuity in transgenic plants." *Nature*, 395: 25.

5. Inose, T. and K. Murata. 1995. "Enhanced Accumulation of Toxic Compound in Yeast Cells Having High Glycolytic Activity: A Case Study on the Safety of Genetically Engineered Yeast." *International Journal of Food Science and Technology*, 30: 141–146.

6. Hansen, Michael, "Genetic Engineering Is Not An Extension of Conventional Plant Breeding," Consumer Policy Institute (January 27, 2000). Submitted to the Food and Drug Administration.

7. Meyer, P., Linn, F., Heidmann, I., Meyer, H., Niedenhof, I., and H. Saedler. 1992. "Endongenous and Environmental Factors Influence 35 S Promoter Methylation of a Maize A1 Gene Construct in Transgenic Petunia and Its Colour Phenotype." *Molecular Genes and Genetics*, 231: 345–352.

8. www.econ.ag.gov/new-at-users

9. Clive James, *International Service for the Acquisition of Agri-Biotech Application, Briefs: Global Review of Commercialized Transgenic Crops, Ithaca, NY, 1998.*

10. *Ag Bio Tech InfoNet at http://www.biotech-info.net/RR_yield_drag_98.pdf*

11. *"ADM Warns Its Grain Suppliers,"* Wall Street Journal, September 2, 1999.

12. "New Genes and Seeds: Protestors in Europe Grow More Passionate," *New York Times,* March 14, 2000.

13. Altieri, Miguel, and Peter Rosset, "Ten Reasons Why Biotechnology Will Not Ensure Food Security, Protect the Environment and Reduce Poverty in the Developing World," Food First/Institute for Food and Development. (October 1999.)

CHAPTER 2

1. *Maclean's* (Jan. 20, 1997) "Science: Unnatural Selection: Are Genetically Altered Foods Really Safe?" A.N. Mayeno and G.J. Gleich "Eosinophilia-Myalgia Syndrome and Tryptophan Production: A Cautionary Tale." *TIBTECH* (1994): 346–352. Phillip Raphals Science (November 2, 1990) "Does Medical Mystery Threaten Biotech?"

2. Ibid.

3. "Why I Cannot Remain Silent: Interview with Dr. Arpad Pusztai" *GM Free* (U.K.) (August–September 1999).

4. Quoted by Joel Bleifuss, "No Small (Genetic) Potatoes," *In These Times* (January 10, 2000).

5. "Cauliflower Mosaic Viral Promoter—A Recipe for Disaster?" *Microbial Ecology in Health and Disease* (no. 4, 1999).

6. "I Was Right, Says GM Row Scientist" (London) *Independent*, March 8, 1999; also sourced by the next footnote, *In These Times*, January 10, 2000.

7. Bleifuss, Joel, "No Small (Genetic) Potatoes, *In These Times* (January 10, 2000). To see the full report by Dr. Pusztai go to www.rri.sari.ac.uk/gmo/index.html

8. Julie Nordless, Steve Taylor et al., "Identification of a Brazil-Nut Allergen in Transgenic Soybeans," *The New England Journal of Medicine*, March 14, 1996.

9. Gladwell, Malcolm, "Biotech Food Products Won't Require Special Rules, FDA Decides." *Washington Post*, May 26, 1992.

10. J. Raloff, "Allergies to this Soy Would Be Nutty," *Science News*, Vol. 149 (March, 16, 1999).

11. Goldburg quote from the book *Imagine a World Without Monarch Butterflies* by Alex Jack, p. 19.

12. Rick Weiss, "Biotech Food Raises a Crop of Questions," *Washington Post* (August 15, 1999).

13. Marian Nestle, "Allergies to Transgenic Foods—Questions of Policy," *The New England Journal of Medicine* (March 14, 1996) pp. 726–27.

14. Legal affidavit submitted August 12, 1998 by Dr. Mae-Wan-Ho in a UK court case on genetically engineered foods. The affidavit is posted on the website of the Institute of Science in Society http://www.i-sis.org/

15. Shiv Chopra and others, rBST (NUTRALAC) "Gaps Analysis" Report By rBST Internal Review Team, Health Protection Branch, Health Canada, April 21, 1998. Also Frederick Bever, "Canadian Agency Questions Approval of Cow Drug by US," Rutland (Vermont) *Herald*, October 6, 1998.

16. Dr. Peter Montague, "Milk rBGH and Cancer," *Rachel's Environment and Health Weekly* #593 (April 9, 1998).

17. The *Milwaukee State Journal* (January 26, 1996).

18. "Study Casts Doubt on Genetically Modified Food," Reuters (January 28, 1999).

19. D.K. Mercer et al., "Fate of Free DNA and Transformation of the Oral Bacterium Streptococcus Gordonii DL1 by Plasmid DNA in NHuman Saliva," *Applied an Environmental Microbiology* 65 (1999): 6–10.

20. Julie Vorman, "Deadly E. Coli Bug May Affect Half of U.S. Cattle," Reuters (November 10, 1999).

21. Mae-Wan Ho, Terje Traavik, et al "Gene Technology & Gene Ecology of Infectious Diseases," *Microbial Ecology in Health and Disease* (Vol. 10): 33–59.

22. For an examination of USDA statistics on pesticide use by U.S. farmers growing herbicide-resistant and Bt crops in 1997–98 see the analysis by Dr. Charles Benbrook, former head of the Agriculture Committee of the National Academy of Sciences at www.biotech-info.net.

23. L. Hardell and M. Erickson, "A Case-Control Study of non-Hodgkin's Lymphoma and Exposure to Pesticides," *Cancer* 86 (6), 1999.

24. Caroline Cox, "Glyphosate, Part I: Toxicology," *Journal of Pesticide Reform*, Fall 1995, Vol. 15 no. 3. See also "Glyphosate, Part 2: Human Exposure and Ecological Effects," *Journal of Pesticide Reform*, Vol. 14 no. 4 (Winter 1995).

25. "Ready for Roundup," GM Free, August/September 1999, Pagell.

26. Marc Lappe and Britt Bailey, *Against the Grain*, (Common Courage Press, 1998), p.147. A. Garcia et al., "Paternal Exposure to Pesticides and Congenital

Malformations," *Scandinavian Journal of Work-Related and Environmental Health* 24 (1998): 473–80.

27. A. Garcia., "Paternal Exposure to Pesticides and Congenital Malformations, " *Scandinavian Journal of Work-Related and Environmental Health* 24:473–80, 1998.

28. Marc Lappe and Britt Bailey, *Against the Grain: Biotechnology and the Corporate Takeover of Your Food* (Common Courage Press, 1998), pp. 41–47.

CHAPTER 3

1. James Kling, "Could Transgenic Crops One Day Breed Superweeds," *Science* 274 (1994): 180–181.

2. Wilson, Graeme, "Farmers told there is no escape from GM pollen," *U.K. Daily Mail* (January 19, 2000).

3. Center for Food Safety, "Greenpeace, Center for Food Safety and Organic Farmers Sue EPA Over Gene-Altered Crops," Press Release (February 18, 1999).

4. L. Hansen and J. Obrycki, "Non-target effects of Bt corn pollen on the Monarch butterfly (Lepidoptera: Danaidae), " Iowa State University, Ames, IA 50011. From: http://www.ent.iastate.edu/entoc/ncb99/prog/abs/D81.html

5. C. Crecchio and G. Stotzky, "Insecticidal Activity and Biodegradation of the Toxin from Bacillus Thuringiensis Subsp.Kurstaki Bound to Humic Acids from the Soil," *Soil Biology and Biochemistry* 30 (1998): 463–70.

6. D. Saxena et al., "Insecticidal Toxin in Root Exudates from Bt Corn," *Nature* 402:480, 1999.

7. Holmes, M.J., Ingham, E.R. "The effects of genetically engineered microorganisms on soil foodwebs," *Bulletin of the Ecological Society of America,* Supplement (1994):75:97.

8. Vandana Shiva, *Biopiracy: The Plunder of Nature and Knowledge* (South End Press, 1997), 34–35.

9. MacArthur, Mary, "Triple-Resistant Canola Weeds Found in Alberta," *Western Producer* (February 10, 2000).

10. *The Times-Picayune,* "Blue Revolution May Be Wave Of Future" (January 16, 2000).

11. Muir WM, Howard RD "Possible ecological risks of transgenic organism release-when transgenes affect mating success: sexual selection and the Trojan gene hypothesis," *PNAS* 96 (1999):13853–56).

12. Associated Press, "New Zealand firm promises to stop breeding 'Frankenfish' " (February 27, 2000).

13. Keith Schneider, "Go Ahead Likely on Crop Tinkering, But Some Are Wary," *The New York Times,* (May 25, 1994).

CHAPTER 4

1. Michael Fox, *Eating with Conscience: The Bioethics of Food,* (NewSage Press, 1997), 76.

2. Research Advancement Foundation International, "AgBiotech's Five Jumbo Gene Giants," Jan. 7, 2000 www.rafi.org>

3. Martin Teitel and Kimberly Wilson, *Genetically Engineered Food: Changing the Nature of Nature*, (Park Street Press, 1999) page 16.

4. Kendall, Peter, "Engineered Crops Face Barren Season, Farmers Fear Controversy Over Genetically Altered Seed May Make Harvest Unmarketable," *Chicago Tribune* (January 24, 2000).

5. General Accounting Office, "Biotechnology—Information on Prices of Genetically Modified Seeds in the United States and Argentina," Washington, D.C., January 2000, p. 10.

6. Fox, J. L. 1997. "Farmers Say Monsanto's Engineered Cotton Drops Bolls." *Nature Biotechnology*, 15: 1233.

7. Hansen, Michael, "Genetic Engineering Is Not An Extension of Conventional Plant Breeding," Consumer Policy Institute (January 27, 2000). Submitted to the Food and Drug Administration.

8. Charles Benbrook, "Evidence of the Magnitude and Consequences of the Round-up Ready Soybean Yield Drag From University-based Varietal Trials in 1998, " July 13, 1999. From www.biotechinfo.net

9. Montague, Peter, "Sustainability and Ag Biotech," *Rachel's Environment & Health Weekly*, #686 (February 10, 2000).

10. American Corn Growers Association, "Corn Growers Complete Survey on Farmer Planting Intentions for Upcoming Growing Season," Press Release (February 21, 2000.)

11. "Family Farmers Warn: If Your Next Crop is GMO, It May Be Your Last," National Family Farm Coalition, (November 23, 1999).

12. National Family Farm Coalition, "Farmers' Declaration on Genetic Engineering in Agriculture" (November 1999).

13. Cochrane, Willard, "A Food and Agricultural Policy for the 21st Century," Institute for Agriculture and Trade Policy (February 2000).

14. Associated Press, "Too Few Farmers Left to Count, Agency Says" (October 10, 1993).

15. Tait, Nikki, "Farmers Ponder Seed Options: Larger U.S. Farms Are Tending to Plant GM Crops While Smaller Concerns Are Looking for a Non-GM Premium," *The Financial Times* (March 7, 2000).

16. Brewster Kneen, *Farmageddon: Food and the Culture of Biotechnology,* (New Society Publishers, 1999).

17. Associated Press, "There Are as Many People Overweight in World as Underfed," (March 5, 2000).

18. Vandana Shiva, *Biopiracy: The Plunder of Nature and Knowledge*, (South End Press, 1997), 20.

19. Andrew Kimbrell, *"Biocolonization,"* *The Case Against the Global Economy*, (Sierra Club Books, 1996), 133.

20. Vandana Shiva, *Biopiracy*, 55.

CHAPTER 5

1. Greenpeace report, *FDA Approved: Genetically Engineered Soy and Corn in Baby Food and Nutritional Supplements* (June 10, 1999).
2. Prince of Wales, "Questions about Genetically Modified Organisms," *The Daily Mail* (June 1, 1999).
3. Center for Food Safety, Lawsuit filed May 27, 1998. Federal Court, Washington, DC.
4. Statement of Rebecca Goldburg, Environmental Defense Fund, At the FDA Public Hearing on Genetically Engineered Foods. November 30, 1999 Washington, DC.
5. Lilliston, Ben, "Aiding and Abetting—U.S. Regulatory System Turns Blind Eye Toward Genetically Engineered Foods" *Multinational Monitor* (January/February 2000).
6. Ibid.
7. Comments from Dr. Linda Kahl, FDA compliance officer, to Dr. James Maryanski, FDA Biotechnology Coordinator, about the Federal Register document "Statement of Policy: Foods from Genetically Modified Plants." Dated January 8, 1992. Can be viewed at: www.biointegrity.org
8. Comments from Dr. Louis J. Pribyl re: the "Biotechnology Draft Document, 2/27/92." Dated March 6, 1992. Can be viewed at: www.biointegrity.org.
9. Associated Press, "Better Study Is Urged Of Biotech Crops' Effects" (February 18, 2000).
10. Center for Food Safety, Lawsuit filed February 18, 1999 against U.S. Environmental Protection Agency. Can be viewed at: www.centerforfoodsafety.org/li/BT2ndam.html.
11. Lilliston, Ben, "Aiding and Abetting—U.S. Regulatory System Turns Blind Eye Toward Genetically Engineered Foods" *Multinational Monitor* (January/February 2000).
12. Goldburg, Rebecca, Environmental Defense Fund. Testimony before the U.S. House of Representatives Committee on Science's Subcommittee on Basic Research (October 1999).
13. Lilliston, Ben, "Aiding and Abetting—U.S. Regulatory System Turns Blind Eye Toward Genetically Engineered Foods," *Multinational Monitor* (January/February 2000).
14. Rick Weiss, "Next Food Fight Brewing Over Listing Genes on Labels." *Washington Post*, August 15, 1999.
15. Food and Drug Administration, "Statement of Policy: Foods Derived From New Plant Varieties," *Federal Register*, Vol. 57. No. 104 (May 29, 1992), 229991.
16. Coca-Cola, November 9, 1999 letter from Kathy Daly, Consumer Affairs Specialist to Debbie Ortman.

CHAPTER 6

1. Union of Concerned Scientists. Updated November 1999. Webpage: www.uscusa.org.

2. Robinson, Claire, "GM Animal Feed: No regulation, no segregation; no choice," Vol. 1 No. 4 of *GM-FREE* (November/December 1999), 4.
3. Mothers for Natural Law, Much of this information can be found at the Mothers for Natural Law website: www.safefood.org.
4. Blythman, Joanna, *How To Avoid GM Foods* (Fourth Estate, London. 1999), 58.
5. Ibid, 61.
6. Ibid, 68–71.
7. *Consumer Reports* (September 1999).
8. Jeff Neff, "The 1999 Top 100 Companies," Thomson Corporation Company and Putman Publishing Company (May 1, 1999).
9. Greenpeace report, *FDA Approved: Genetically Engineered Soy and Corn in Baby Food and Nutritional Supplements* (June 10, 1999).
10. Scott Kilman, "USA: Monsanto's Biotech Spud Is Being Pulled from the Fryer at Fast-Food Chain," *Wall Street Journal* (April 28, 2000).
11. "McCain blows cool on GM potatoes," *Farmer's Weekly* (December 3, 1999.)

CHAPTER 7

1. Chase, Brett. "Whole Foods, Wild Oats Chains to Ban Gene-Altered Ingredients," Bloomberg News Service (December 30, 1999).
2. Lagnado, Lucette, "Gerber Baby Food, Grilled by Greenpeace, Plans Swift Overhaul," *Wall Street Journal* (July 30, 1999).
3. Scott Kilman, "USA: Monsanto's Biotech Spud Is Being Pulled from the Fryer at Fast-Food Chain, " *Wall Street Journal* (April 28, 2000).
4. Kilman, Scott. "Biotech Scare Sweeps Europe, and Companies Wonder If U.S. Is Next," *Wall Street Journal* (October 7, 1999).
5. Ibid.
6. "Seagram Co. Tells Farmers It Won't Buy Genetically Modified Corn," *Toronto Star* (February 9, 2000).
7. Jack, Alex. *Imagine a World Without Monarch Butterflies*. One Peaceful World Press (2000).
8. Laura's Lean Beef Web site: www.laurasleanbeef.com.
9. Greenpeace Press Release. December 20, 1999. "U.K. Supermarkets Move Out of GM-fed Animal Products. U.K.'s largest retailer, Tesco, pulling out in 2000."
10. Monsanto. "Status Update Regarding: Posilac® Bovine Somatotropin," December 10, 1999. Can be found on their Web site: www.monsanto.com
11. Teitel, Martin, and Kimberly Wilson. *Genetically Engineered Food: Changing the Nature of Nature* (Park Street Press, 1999), 35.
12. E-mail from Jennifer K. DeClue, R.D., Nutrition Specialist, Office of Consumer Affairs, Purina (January 5, 2000).

CHAPTER 8

1. John Fetto, "Home on the Organic Range," *American Demographics* (August 1999).
2. Organic Trade Association. Business Facts. Webpage: www.ota.com.
3. Merrill, Ann. "Organics Go Mainstream," *Minneapolis Star Tribune* (September 8, 1999).
4. Lau, Edie, "A Worried Public Turns to Organic Foods: Research Funds, Once Scarce, May See an Upturn," *Sacramento Bee Science Writer* (February 23, 2000).
5. Anderson, Jens-Otto, "Farming, Plant Nutrition and Food Quality," Presentation to the Soil Association (January 3, 2000.) Also, BBC News, "Organic Food 'Proven' Healthier," (January 3, 2000).
6. Long, Cheryl. "Open Letter to the USDA," *Organic Gardening Magazine* (November/December 1999).
7. Ibid.
8. Kinney, Donal. "Southwest Cooperative Grocers Association Meets in Albuquerque," *Co-op Connection*. Albuquerque, NM.
9. Sustainable Agriculture Research and Education (SARE) Program, January 5, 2000 Press Release, "New Directory Links Farmers, Consumers in Food Partnerships."
10. Ludwig, Oliver, "Farmers Markets Sprout Up Across America," *Reuters* (September 1999).
11. Lagnado, Lucette. "U.S. Restaurants Try To End Genetically Modified Food," *The Wall Street Journal* (March 9, 2000).